LICENSED TO DRILL

Dentist on the Loose!

by

Barrie Lawrence

**Grosvenor House
Publishing Limited**

The right of Barrie Lawrence to be identified as the author of this
work has been asserted by him in accordance with Section 78
of the Copyright, Designs and Patents Act 1988

The book cover picture is copyright to Derek Blois
Cover design by Derek Blois

This book is published by
Grosvenor House Publishing Ltd
Link House
140 The Broadway, Tolworth, Surrey, KT6 7HT.
www.grosvenorhousepublishing.co.uk

A CIP record for this book
is available from the British Library

ISBN 978-1-78623-841-2

This book is dedicated with much love, affection and gratitude, to my parents, Brenda and the late Dick Lawrence, without whose support and encouragement, I would almost certainly never have been *licensed to drill.*

Other books by Barrie Lawrence

Light autobiographical

A DENTIST'S STORY   Grosvenor House Publishing (2014)

PATIENTS FROM HEAVEN –
and Other Places!   Grosvenor House Publishing (2015)

Christian

THERE MUST BE MORE TO LIFE THAN THIS!
                          New Wine Publishing (2012)

THE CURIOUS CASE OF THE CONSTIPATED CAT
                          Grosvenor House Publishing (2016)

Contents

Foreword

"Come on, Barrie - you can't have *more* stories from your dental days. Can you? Honestly?"

Well, the answer is a resounding Yes! So, having written two books of light dental banter, why write another? And more than banter. Let me briefly explain.

Firstly, the more I write, the more I am asked to speak. And from time to time, this triggers memories of amusing incidents that I had previously forgotten. These incidents accumulate, furnishing me with more and more *material*

The second reason is very simple, in that people keep asking me, "When is your next book coming out?"

Thirdly, I did not really set out to write even *one* book. I have now written five, of which three are light, dental anecdotal. I have noticed, however, that some authors produce a *trilogy*. To me, there is something of a completeness about a trilogy. So here is my third offering on this subject, and, if it is a trilogy, probably my last. But having said that, I have read somewhere that one should never say 'Never again!"

Finally, I enjoy writing. I was ten years of age when I entered an essay competition on the subject of 'Wroxham', which was the name of the village where I lived at that time. I enthusiastically spent an hour or two with my fountain pen and a couple of sheets of A4 paper - and won. At University, I had a satirical column in a glossy magazine, *The London Hospital Gazette.* I wrote under the pen name of Tweedledum, but also had poetry published under my own name. Since then, I have had various articles, usually on the lighter side of dentistry, published in magazines and suchlike. But I never really contemplated writing a book.

And then the practice's favourite patient, Prof. Toby Lewis, started giving me that rather mischievous smile of his, as he said, "Write a book, Barrie." He would join my wife and I for lunch, and be just a little more pressing. I will not be further tedious - I wrote a book. And then others.

* * *

For many years, I was a great James Bond *aficionado*. I am not quite sure how it happened, as, having been raised in the depths of rural Norfolk in the UK, I arrived at London University in 1963 in a state of profound naivety.

"*Dr. No* is on at a cinema locally," said one of my fellow students at The London Hospital Medical College. *Dr. No?* I had occasionally seen *Dr. Kildare* on my parents' small black and white television set, and *Emergency - Ward 10* had been a familiar title to me. But *Dr. No?* I was not really interested.

Most of my fellow students were more than eager to see this '*James Bond*' film. James Bond? Even in the backwaters of agricultural England, I had heard of Gregory Peck, Clark Gable and John Wayne. But James Bond? However, I decided to keep my friends company at the local Odeon.

It was electrifying! I was riveted to the screen as 007 wrestled, punched, and shot his way to the victorious climax, where the villain was finally and decisively disposed of. And Bond won the heart of Honey Rider, played by an actress named in my *Private Eye* magazine as 'Ursula Undress'.

I bought all the Bond books that had been published at that time, and read them at least three times apiece. I was mortified when Ian Fleming collapsed and died of a heart attack in 1964. He was only fifty-six, but he drank and smoked liked the immortal Bond. Two more books were published, and the films continue to be made to this day. I was one of the first to the cinema as each one was released. I bought the videos, and later the DVDs. My wife and I could recite the lines ahead of the actors, and for a while, purely coincidentally, I drove a white Lotus Esprit almost identical to the one Bond himself drove in the latest movie at that time – *The Spy Who Loved Me (1977)*.

It was shortly after this that I realised that the long number on my dental practice credit card was significant. It ended in 006. I would never be licensed to kill by Her Majesty's Secret Service, but, in a manner of speaking, Her Majesty's National Health Service had given me a *licence to drill*. Or, to be strictly factual, the Royal College of Surgeons of England had furnished me with such a licence back in 1969.

For many years, I have been an after-dinner speaker for a variety of societies, organisations and political parties. Also for the Women's Institute non-dinner meetings, and similar. Additionally, I speak at evangelistic fellowships, such as the Full Gospel Businessmen, where I have been president in Norwich for the past five years. For the latter, my remit is to tell the story of my spiritual journey, though I have to be myself, and humour is liable to creep in. But for my secular speeches, humour is expected, and can indeed abound - though I do mention that I am a born-again Christian, and that there will be no smut. Ladies and children are quite safe when I am speaking.

So I trust that you will find humour, as well as facts - interesting, fascinating and almost unbelievable perhaps - concerning the history of dentistry, and the naked truth concerning what goes on behind the closed surgery door of a dental practice. I trust that you will be filled with amusement and amazement at these painfully fascinating extractions from my life as a dental surgeon - a time when I was *licensed to drill*.

Barrie Lawrence
Frettenham, Norfolk, UK.
November 2016

Introduction

The name was Bond. James Bond. 007. I have no idea when my hero received his licence to kill, but I was given my *licence to drill* in mid-December 1968. At last, I was a dentist on the loose – and almost immediately went into active service!

* * *

"Barrie Lawrence has qualified!" exclaimed Dudley Farmer. He banged his near-empty pint of best bitter down onto the bar, with a resounding thud that commanded the attention of all present. The buzz of conversation around the bar in the Sammie, colloquial name for the Good Samaritan Public House, much-loved, and patronised almost exclusively by staff and students at The London Hospital in Whitechapel, came to an abrupt halt. Every eye was on Dudley, who appeared dazed and in a state of shock.

"Lawrence has qualified?" he exclaimed again, as if looking for confirmation from someone other than the grinning dental student who had just brought the news. "That's like letting a monkey loose with a pistol."

Laughter exploded from the gathered throng of students and ricocheted around the bar. But it was a nine-minute wonder, and Dudley's mug was soon full again as the evening continued.

* * *

Meanwhile, the monkey was well away from the hilarity in the Sammie, and the facetious remarks of Dudley Farmer, Senior Registrar and lecturer in Dental Surgery. Dudley liked to be known as one of the lads, could drink most other chaps under the table, and regularly lost his trousers at formal dinners after loudly challenging those present, "Debag me if you can!"

The monkey with the pistol? He was actually with his fiancée at the best Indian restaurant in London. Oblivious to the banter back in Whitechapel, he enjoyed the salute from the beturbanned seven-foot Asian doorman, who led them to the lift. Stepping out at the first floor was like re-entering India in all its Victorian colonial splendour. Another beturbanned gentleman showed them to a bar, and later to a table where the high-backed wooden chairs each had 'VR' carved in the top cross strut, and where the colour of each turban denoted the function of the gentleman wearing it; barman, hors d'hoevre waiter, wine waiter and so forth. One could indeed be back in the days of the Raj. It was not until the following morning that I was informed that I was now akin to a monkey with a pistol.

* * *

"It's 006. Licensed to drill," I said in a voice that I hoped would sound both suave, and - lethal!

"Oh, it's you," said the young lady on the other end of the telephone. "And I'm Moneypenny."

"Okay," I replied. "The name's Lawrence. Barrie Lawrence. I'm getting a little low on *ammo*, so stand by for my order."

Ten years had passed, and I was ordering dental supplies for my multi-surgeried dental practice in the city of Norwich. I could hear Audrey, the receptionist at Porro's, pick up a pen, and I duly reeled off my order for ammo - 4 boxes of dental amalgam in capsule form ("the ones that look like *bullets*"), 5 boxes of *cartridges* for my anaesthetic syringe... And having completed the order, I recited my credit card details, where the long number ended in 006.

"006. Licensed to drill. I love it," said Audrey. "You going off on any adventures soon?"

"This very afternoon," I answered. "Goldentooth!"

* * *

This conversation, and variations on it, would take place on a monthly basis when I telephoned one of our dental supply companies to restock with various consumables. It was after I had changed my credit card and was reading out the latest long number, that the final three digits caught my attention. 006. I was an avid fan of Ian Fleming's character, James Bond, having read each of the books several times, and enjoyed the films as they came out over the years. Even if Roger Moore was a bit too silly at times. And even though George Lazenby was perhaps, rather wooden. Only Sean Connery really *was* James Bond, of course. And as for those after Moore and Connery had stood down..... though Daniel Craig probably fitted the bill best.

I watched all the videos with my wife, and after a few times through, we were coming out with the lines before the characters did themselves. Then my wife left me to marry a man she had met on the Internet, and when that marriage failed, she married yet again, having found - James Bond. And I am not joking - she really did meet and marry a James Bond. I wish her well, as I recall the days when we worked together, visiting housebound patients in my white Lotus Esprit, just like the one that Roger Moore drove at the time in the Bond movie, *The Spy Who Loved Me* (1977).

* * *

Licensed to drill? It had been back in December 1968 when, having taken my final examinations after five years of dental training at the London Hospital, I caught the Tube to Russell Square underground station and strolled along to Senate House. The results would be posted there mid-morning, and I was not surprised to find a few other anxious-looking students hovering around, and trying to make light of what we all really knew was a very serious business. Today, no doubt, students sit by their computer screens, but this was well before the Internet was up and running in its present form.

I gave a sigh of relief as I saw my name on the sheet posted on the board, and quickly broke into a broad grin. I had qualified. After more than five years of drilling, filling, injecting, extracting, straightening and studying, studying, studying, I was now a dental surgeon. Well, to most people, 'dentist'.

News travels fast at times. That same evening saw the announcement in the bar at the Sammie, prompting Dudley Farmer's almost predictable response

I suppose I was fairly prominent amongst the students, not because I had excelled on the rugby field or even academically, but because I had been there a little longer than most. I had failed an earlier exam, twice, and had taken an extra year to qualify. In my earlier years, I had over-indulged in beer drinking. So had most of my fellow students, but I was a joker with it. I also wrote satire, under the pen name *Tweedledum*, in *The London Hospital Gazette*. And having been high profile as a beer-drinking comedian, I then had a Damascus Road experience and became a born-again Christian. I was no evangelist, but I wanted everybody to know of my life-changing experience, and that they too needed to accept Christ as their Saviour and Lord. Not everybody wanted to know that, and not everybody was amused - yet everyone seemed to know Barrie Lawrence. Dudley Farmer certainly did.

But, licensed to drill, I was now on the loose. Where would I go, and what would I do? A monkey with a pistol? It had certainly caused an explosion of unbridled mirth in the bar at the Sammie that evening, but I was unaware of it, having taken my fiancée to The Veeraswamy, that Indian restaurant in Swallow Street in the centre of London, where we celebrated in style.

I could not know that within six months a patient would leap from my dental chair and flee the surgery, hotly pursued through the town by Yours Truly, white coat flapping out behind me as we sprinted along the streets of Shaftesbury in Dorset. Well, I was young, and nobody had told me that dental surgeons were *not* supposed to chase patients who legged it out of the surgery. Nor was I to know that another patient, a professional man in a very smart suit, would push me aside as he made a break for it, crashing out through the door of the practice to collapse in the long dew-sodden grass of the practice's back lawn. And later, back in my home county of Norfolk at my Norwich practice, a young man would leap from the chair, career out through the surgery door and virtually tumble down the stairs leading to the front door. I did not need to chase him, as his big brother said, "I'll get 'im mate," and crashed out after him, felling him with a rugby tackle outside the fruit and veg shop on the corner, and bringing him back in a terrible state.

Generally my relationship with patients was good, amiable, and relaxed, but there was that 006 on my credit card, and there were those words spoken by Dudley Farmer back in the students' bar when I qualified. So, ever happy to laugh at myself, and a few other members of my profession, and not least colleagues who worked with me over the years (whilst maintaining anonymity for those who *did* behave like monkeys with pistols), I have brought together a collection of stories from my years in dental practice. There are chapters with stories of Heroes (patients we were particularly fond of), Villains (patients that we found a trifle challenging) and Memorable Others (patients worthy of a mention because they were simply 'different'). I have changed names and details in order to preserve anonymity for those who were foolish, bad, or who simply acted as though demented. Patients *and* dentists. And there were those patients that the staff loved, amongst whom was the private detective we called Hammer (after the character immortalised by the author Mickey Spillane). "Use my real name," he said when I showed him the manuscript. I had changed his name to something like John Smith. "The name's Clarke. Phillip Clarke. Use it."

I hope you enjoy reading some of the escapades of nearly forty years of dental practice. But I would not read this book before visiting your local practitioner. He too, you see, is licensed to drill. He too, could be a monkey with a pistol – 'a dentist on the loose'.

PART ONE

INTO ACTION!

Chapter 1

Licensed to Drill.

Louis Thurston – 'Lou' to his friends - was out on a drinking spree with some of his mates.

"You might be a good dentist," said Izzy, "But my roots are so long that the last dentist I went to 'ad to give up. I just 'ad to suffer."

"Yer think I couldn't get 'em art? Don't you Adam and Eve it," said Lou, using the rhyming cockney slang he had been brought up with in the East End of London. "I can get *any* teef art."

An hour passed, along with several further pints of ale, and both Lou and his friend Izzy were in fierce, alcohol-fuelled dispute. Izzy maintained that no dentist - absolutely *no* dentist - could budge his molar teeth, whilst Lou prided himself on being able to remove any tooth. *ANY* tooth.

And so it was that midnight saw the two men laughing, cursing, and stumbling to Lou's surgery in the heart of Cockney London. There was a wager by this time. £5 said Lou could not remove any of Izzy's molars, and £5 said he could. His surgery resembled a scaled down medieval torture chamber, with forceps that had seen better days, and a rather menacing drill hanging from the ceiling.

"Just the one," said Izzy, settling somewhat warily in Lou's cast-iron dental chair. Lou brought huge straps out from the back of the chair, and Izzy was soon helplessly bound to its frame. (Years later, in a similar scene, Laurence Olivier would

3

ask Dustin Hoffman, "Is it safe?" Those readers who have seen the film *Marathon Man* will know exactly what I am referring to, and if of a nervous disposition, will shudder. Why did my most apprehensive patients sit and watch that film the evening before an appointment, and walk in looking like Dustin Hoffman at the end of that most memorable scene?)

Izzy was almost in a coma due to the ale, and looked as though he had received a general anaesthetic. Lou's judgement was seriously impaired as he approached the unfortunate victim.

"Open yer marf then," slurred Lou. Izzy regained partial consciousness, and opened his mouth. The beaks of the forceps sliced through the gum around one of Izzy's upper molars, and there was a delayed drunken 'shcream' as bone was forced away from tooth.

"Help!" was muffled to a large extent, partly by ale-paralysis and partly from Izzy's mouth being full of hand and forceps. But with a mighty wrench, Lou leapt back, molar gripped firmly in the beaks of his forceps.

"So I can't get yer teef art of yer marf?" said Lou. "Well I'll b*****y show yer what I can do." And without further ado, he dived back into Izzy's mouth, oblivious to blood forming small rivulets from the corners, and dripping off his victim's chin.

"See," shouted Lou with drunken abandon, as a second molar was extracted with great gusto. "And another... and another...." - and Lou, with manic hilarity, attacked one tooth after another, until Izzy's entire dentition lay in a bloody heap in an enamel bowl.

"And that's a fiver, me ole cock, cos yer lost yer wager," he announced triumphantly. Izzy woefully produced a five pound note, and lurched out through the door on his way home, whilst Lou staggered up the stairs to the flat over the surgery.

* * *

Bang! Bang! Bang! Lou's head was pounding as he was woken from his drunken slumber by another pounding.

"Go away," he shouted. "I'm closed."

"Closed. *CLOSED?* Yer'll come darn here now. *NOW!* What 'ave you done to my Izzy? You're a bastard, Thurston, that's what you are," screamed Izzy's wife Huldah.

And so it was that Lou stumbled down his 'apple and pears', (Cockney for stairs) and opening his surgery door, was confronted by Izzy's enraged wife.

"Yer'll pay for this, yer drunken scumbag," hissed Huldah. "Yer pulled all 'is teef art, yer did. Scumbag. Yer'll pay for this. Look at 'im. Yer'll make 'im new teef, yer will. And yer won't charge 'im."

This could be quite a long story - and it's a true story - but suffice to say that Lou sobered up eventually and made false teeth, for free, for his former mate, Izzy. That was around the year 1920, when anyone could become a dentist. In fact, even Lou could, who was largely self-taught, and quite good at it. But change was in the air, sadly for Lou. He told me the story himself years later, in 1969, when he worked as a dental technician at the practice in Shaftesbury where I first practised after qualifying. Let me complete Lou's story.

* * *

Lou had been born and bred in the East End of London, and as he approached school leaving age, in his mid-teens, needed to find work. He had once visited a dentist, and was intrigued by the practitioner's dexterity in removing a tooth. He enquired around the area, and was successful in finding a dentist who would take him on as an apprentice. He watched, he listened, he sometimes 'had a go', and as soon as the opportunity presented, he rented a small property where he could extract (and occasionally fill) teeth, whilst living in a flat over the surgery.

There were dental schools, but they were the province of the wealthy, ex-public school boys, who then went on to practice in more prestigious, and lucrative, locations. Lou practised for a few years in the East End of London, and when he heard that dentists would have to register if they wanted to continue to practice, decided to ignore it. But the Dentists Act was passed by Parliament in 1921, and those wishing to continue working as dentists, had to pay an annual registration fee of £5. Lou continued to ignore it. The result? A summons to appear at Bow Street Magistrates Court. He was fined £5, and warned that the consequences would be more serious if he continued to practise without registering annually for £5.

"I wasn't going to pay £5 a year to be a dentist," Lou told me. "It seemed a lot of money in them days, though I wish now that I'd paid up. So I became a dental technician, and later moved to Dorset. And here I am."

He was a decent old boy, then in his 70s and working several hours a week to supplement his pension. He had been a rogue, regularly getting drunk and knowing how to handle himself when in a corner. He was a mean, unhappy man. One day he heard the gospel - the Bible message that Jesus changes peoples' lives. He didn't tell me how, but he felt convicted that he needed to surrender his life to Jesus, and found that 'everything changed'. He became a different man in many ways, and when I met him at the practice in Dorset, he was a staunch member of the local Baptist church, and a pillar of the community. Well, that is what Jesus does for people. He changed my life, by changing me, back in October 1965, so I knew what Lou was talking about.

Licensed to drill? It cost £5 a year in 1921, and Lou felt it was not worth it. I suppose, strictly speaking, it was 'registered to drill', but the licence was already an alternative. The 1858 Medical Act had granted the Royal College of Surgeons the power to hold examinations to test the fitness of individuals to practice dentistry. This they did from 1860, and those passing the examinations they set received the qualification LDS. Licence in Dental Surgery - *licence* to drill, so to speak.

Later, universities ran degree courses at dental schools, and those completing the course and passing the examinations were awarded a degree, BDS. Bachelor of Dental Surgery. I trained at the London Hospital in Whitechapel, and was awarded my degree, BDS, by London University in December 1968, receiving the actual piece of paper from Her Majesty, the Queen Mother, in May 1969. I walked stiffly across the podium at the Royal Albert Hall, turned slightly towards the esteemed lady, gave a little bow, and promptly exited stage left.

Later that year, I returned to London, and sat further examinations at the Royal College of Surgeons of England in Lincoln's Inn Fields. As a result, I was awarded a Licence in Dental Surgery. It was a parallel qualification to my degree, but it gave me several more letters after my name. BDS LDS RCSE - Bachelor of Dental Surgery, Licence in Dental Surgery, Royal College of Surgeons of England. Some people travelled significant distances to my Norwich city practice, as apparently I had more letters after my name than any other dentist in the 'Yellow Pages' of the telephone directory in the county of Norfolk. But it did not mean I was any better than the other dentists. In fact, you might say that it simply meant - I was *licensed to drill!*

Chapter 2

Shaken, Not Stirred

Shaken? My eyes opened like tea plates and my hair would have stood a foot high if it had not been for the tight blond curls.

"The shrieks were deafening, even though they came from the next building," said my father as we sat round the tea table, enjoying - well, we *had* been enjoying - bread and butter with my mother's homemade strawberry jam, and the fruit cake she had baked earlier that day. "Everybody could hear it, and then there were cries of 'Snookums is after me! Snookums is after me!' They must have been giving someone gas. They should never have let the dentist work next door to us."

"Dick! Can't you see that Barrie is terrified?" exclaimed my mother. "You know he is seeing the dentist there tomorrow."

My father had, at times, an unfortunate sense of humour, and there are times when I think I have inherited it.

We were living in the small town of Wroxham on the Norfolk broads. Having been born in Norfolk, and lived there for my first 3 days, my mother had left the nursing home and returned over the county border to Bungay, Suffolk where she lived in the family home over the business. Another year or two and my father returned from the war, and we moved to Hertfordshire. But 1953 saw us arrive back in Norfolk, where my father worked in Barclays Bank - next to the dentist!

* * *

Sugar had no more to do with dental decay than inhaling ciga-rette smoke had to do with lung cancer in those days. We had been living in the small Hertfordshire village of Barkway for six years when, on 5th February 1953, a government announce-ment had the community buzzing with excitement. Sweets were no longer rationed. My parents obtained a large circular tin and immediately filled it with various goodies from the confec-tioners across the road from our home. I was supposed to ask first, but the sweets were readily available from that tin kept just behind the sideboard doors. Before long I had toothache.

There was a conference of whispered voices in the kitchen of my grandparents' home, in Peterborough, where we were spending the weekend. I was not particularly interested in what the grown-ups were talking about. "Dentist", and 'gas', and 'have it out' were not words or phrases that I understood; they were grown-up talk. Boring. I went and played in the garden, oblivious to my grandfather making a telephone call. And then I was called indoors.

"We're going into the city," said my father. "There's a man there who will make your tooth better."

The man was Mr. Matthews. They led me up the garden path, my father rang the doorbell, and we entered the building. Not only was the hallway dark, but there was an unpleasant odour hanging in the air. Not nice. Our footsteps echoed from the linoleum flooring, and a rather stern looking lady showed us into a room with upright chairs around the walls. There were a few people sitting there, and they all looked sad. Silence. It reminded me of the church that my other grandparents took us to when we stayed with them. Everyone was silent, and stared through whatever wall faced them. Perhaps we were allowed to whisper, like they did in my other grandparents' church.

"What are we doing?" I whispered to my mother.

"He won't be long," she answered in hushed reverential tones. "He'll make your tooth better."

We sat and stared at the wall opposite us. Just a wall. "Fred Bloggins," said the stern lady now standing in the doorway.

The portly man with the red face stood up and solemnly followed her out of the room, and we could hear their footsteps echoing into the distant recesses of the building. We stared at the walls.

"Ethel White," said the poker-faced lady with the matching voice. Fred Bloggins could be heard leaving through the front door, as Ethel traipsed submissively into the void. We stared at the walls.

"Barrie Lawrence," said the voice. My father stood up, and somewhat awkwardly took my hand as we followed Miss Stern along a lengthy corridor.

It was a strange room indeed. The main feature was a heavy, gaunt cast-iron chair standing starkly in the centre of the room. There was a very worn, faded, tan-coloured cushion and backrest - and that odour. Clinical. Acrid. Unforgettable. Grey cabinets lined the walls, and stainless steel dishes, and a large jar with metal dart-like objects suspended in a pale yellow liquid stood on the work-surfaces.

My father and Mr. Matthews whispered together, after which my father shot me an uncomfortable glance before leaving the room. Panic. I looked round, but there was no escape, as I realised that Miss Stern was now standing in front of the closed door, and another rather solid, deadpan warder was moving in from my left.

Suddenly, arms reached out and pinned me to the back of the chair, as a black rubber mask was placed over my face. More panic. Struggle. Shout. Pinioned by the Peterborough Gestapo, and fighting for my life, I was engulfed in stifling darkness and passed out into... oblivion.

"Spit. Spit it out." There was the sensation of cold, crisp air on my face as, supported under my armpits, my feet dragged behind me and I became aware of roses lining the same garden path that I had been led up an hour earlier.

"Spit. Spit the blood out." My father's instructions ensured a great season for roses in Mr. Matthew's front garden that year.

Shaken? I was shaken, but - an inclination to become a dentist myself? No way. I was shaken, but certainly not stirred to set my sights on the dental profession.

* * *

"Where do you keep your sweet-tin?" I would ask aunts, uncles, friends, and neighbours when we visited their homes. Some did not have a sweet-tin, which caused me to think them rather peculiar. *Everybody* should have a sweet-tin.

Later that year we moved to Wroxham - and again I developed toothache. My father enquired locally, and found that a dentist's surgery was next to the bank where he worked. Had he not heard the shrieks? An appointment was made.

Mr. Henderson-Russell. With a name like that, surely he would be expensive! But with a name like that, surely he would be good! I had a few fillings. The injections made me cry and the drill rumbled away for an eternity. I was relieved to get home, and found comfort in the sweet-tin.

Some months later I yet again developed toothache. Mr. Henderson-Russell had moved, and there was a new man working there. He had an exceptionally high forehead, and my father said that he must have a very large brain and be extremely intelligent. Probably expensive too. Apparently my first molars were deeply decayed, and removing them was not only necessary but would help make room for wisdom teeth one day. If I had any. To quote the comedian Tony Hancock, the needles were like drain pipes coming at me. Shaken? I cried. Cried? I shrieked. My screams must have resonated around Barclays Bank next door. Eventually I left the surgery biting on blood-clotting gauze, and was on my way home. Deeply upset and traumatised - indeed, shaken - I found solace in the much loved sweet-tin.

* * *

I was just entering my teens as we moved eight miles or so to North Walsham, where my father now worked in that community's bank. A new dentist was the talk of the town, and before long I was booked in to see Mr. Charles Pitt-Steele. Red trousers with pink silk shirt, and a gold medallion swinging round his neck together with a breezy manner, caused him to stand out in our small market town. The ladies swooned at the very mention of his name. He was indeed, the talk of the town. He sang like a lark around the surgery, and greeted everyone as an old friend as he strode through the market place. He talked to me as though he was my uncle. He rubbed ointment on the gum before he injected. He used new fine disposable needles, and he was gentle. He had 'the new drill' that made a whistling sound and did not vibrate. And he sang!

* * *

"What are you going to do when you grow up?" was a recurring question at that time. I had read some Freud, which seemed to make sense to me, and thought I might like to become a psychoanalyst. But my passion was catching mice under hay-stacks, and taking them home for breeding. Alongside the frog, the snake, the leeches.... My mother recently told my wife that I always was a difficult child!

Today I reflect on my childhood and the agonies of dental treatment in those early years, contrasted with the style of 'Sandy' Pitt-Steele. Perhaps it was the fact that in Sandy's surgery, I was no longer shaken, but in fact stirred to consider whether maybe I myself might become a dentist one day. Then there was a Career's Exhibition in Peterborough, where I picked up a beautiful booklet with such a tasteful olive green cover, *DENTISTRY - A CAREER AND A FUTURE*. The author was Mr. Neil Livingstone-Ward – with a name like that, my parents would have suspected he was expensive, but good. A few years later he was to teach me dentistry at the London Hospital, where I also discovered that fellow senior members of staff there called him Hank. Hank?

So, whereas those earlier dentists had left me seriously shaken, Sandy Pitt-Steele saw me stirred to consider dentistry as a career. Not shaken, but stirred. Maybe I could be a kind dentist, and not a fearsome man in a white coat. Maybe. Just maybe.

* * *

But there were to be years of study, adventures, hard work, mishaps, surprises and humour before I was eventually licensed to drill. And one of the first things I had to learn at dental school, was how to be a tooth sleuth – which led to a few of those surprises!

Chapter 3

Tooth Sleuth

"Your teeth are fine. No cavities, no extractions, no scaling – in fact, no treatment at all required. Your teeth appear to be in perfect order." I said to the lady sitting in my dental chair. She looked puzzled, and said, "I should think so too," and putting her hand in her mouth, extracted... both upper and lower dentures.

* * *

Every dentist has to learn to check teeth when training at dental school, and there is a limit to how much one can learn from books and in lectures. So, much of the course is hands-on, and in Whitechapel in 1965, those of us who had started out together eighteen months previously, were presented with a varied batch of around thirty patients. Some were young children with their first teeth erupting, while others were approaching their teen years, and starting to need fillings. Other patients of all ages required extractions, gum surgery, crowns, root treatments, bridges and dentures. But every patient needed their teeth examining before any treatment could even be planned.

And so it was that a lady in late middle-age and of few words, walked into the clinic one morning, sat in my dental chair, leaned back and opened her mouth. I was young. I was inexperienced. I had not checked many teeth before. Every tooth looked perfect, and furthermore, my probe slid around each surface without sticking, clicking, catching, or grating. So

I told her that the teeth were fine, and had the surprise of my life when she put her hand to her mouth and extracted the lot - teeth, gums and palate. I caught my breath and was unusually quick thinking as I said, "Well, that just shows you how very natural your false teeth are, fooling even me. They must have been extremely expensive, and I congratulate you on having been to a most excellent dentist." The patient sat and beamed, and I suspected that I had gained a new friend.

I had a similar experience in some ways, many years later, when the denture technician put a lady's new false teeth in a bag with a different patient's name on it. So the teeth in the bag with *her* name on it were not hers, but I was not to know.

"Here are your new teeth," I said with a smile. She removed the existing set, and I popped the new ones in. Clank, clank, click, cough, splutter, spit, shout. "They're too big. They're enormous. They hurt. They're digging in."

A cursory glance told me what had happened, and I took the king-sized dentures out of her mouth and put them on one side to be sterilised. "A trifle on the large size, and feeling absolutely huge because the mouth is so very sensitive. But I think I know what to do, and they will soon be fitting a treat," I hastened to explain.

I raced down the stairs to reception, where dentures from the laboratory were stored, awaiting fitting. A quick look through the assortment revealed the real teeth for the patient sitting in the chair.

Back in the surgery, I handed them to the patient, with a "Just try them now!" She did, and flashing her brand new smile at me, asked, "However did you do that?"

"Just 5 minutes in our new shrinking solution," I replied.

"Oh, you are a clever man," said one satisfied patient.

* * *

One of the first things we were taught at dental school was how to examine the teeth and gums. Sitting in the chair, the patient is generally unaware of exactly what is going on in their mouth.

Are the teeth healthy? Are the fillings sound? Are the gums healthy? I once went to have my teeth checked by a young dentist, who spent around 90 seconds in my mouth, and whose probe actually touched just three teeth. Did he not know I was a dentist myself? I did not go back to see him again.

I was a tooth sleuth! It was my job to seek out that which was bad - and eliminate it. I had been taught the basics whilst training, but along the way one learns a few further lessons. So what should you expect from a dental examination, generally known as a 'check-up'?

Firstly, I would ask the patient if all was well. Although the usual response was that they were not experiencing any problems, there were predictably those people who either had pain, an ache, sensitivity, a sharp edge, a loose tooth, or some similar problem that they hoped I could resolve. And on occasions, there would be a challenge - or a surprise.

"My teeth itch," said a middle-aged, rather shabbily dressed lady from a local housing development.

"Itch?" I enquired. "Could you tell me more about it please?"

"Itch. They itch. I want to scratch them, cos they just keep itching. They're driving me mad, they are."

That was a challenge indeed, because there was no indication of decay either clinically (looking at them and probing them) or radiographically (X-rays). So what does one do? I scaled and polished them - but they itched. I sent her to the dental hygienist - but they itched. I applied a desensitising varnish - they still itched. It seemed that nothing would stop the teeth itching.

Then the patient lost confidence in me, and found a dentist who would take radical, decisive action that would surely resolve the problem. The teeth were extracted, after which the lady lost confidence in that dentist and retuned to me.

"It's my gums. They itch. Where the teeth used to be - my gums itch."

There comes a point at which one passes the buck.

"This is a very difficult and unusual condition that you have, Mrs. Thompson," I explained. "You need to see a specialist, as

I really feel this is beyond my understanding. I will refer you to the local hospital."

Maybe it was a coward's way out, but what else was I to do? Maybe, just perhaps, the consultant in oral surgery might have the answer, or more likely would pass her on to the periodontist, or endodontist - or psychiatrist. And at every stage in her journey, I could imagine each successive consultant exclaiming, "Itch. *Itch*? What do you mean - itch?"

On another occasion a young man sat in my chair, and when asked if he had any problems with his teeth replied, "No mate. No problems. Everything is A OK." And he gave me a thumbs-up to emphasise that all was well.

He had a somewhat furtive look about him, peering at me out of the corner of his eye as I washed my hands, and he even seemed to open his mouth rather reluctantly as I approached with mirror and probe.

All was well? He was 'A OK'? Thumbs-up? Then what was this large dark abyss in his lower left first molar. I told him that without needing to use my probe, I could clearly see a large cavity in a molar tooth.

"B*gger!" he exclaimed, pushing my hands out of his mouth, and sitting upright in the chair. "B*gger! I *thought* you'd find that one." And with resignation, he laid back in the chair and opened his mouth again.

It was a game? If I found the cavity, he was disappointed. And if I had told him that I could see nothing wrong...

* * *

A general look around the mouth will make one aware of any obvious problems, such as a large cavity, a fractured cusp, an ulcer on the gum and suchlike. This examination may seem cursory, but will leave the dentist informed with regard to any obvious, gross problem, but one does need to go further. Maybe I should have explained this to my young colleague who took under ninety seconds and touched three teeth.

My second step was to dry the teeth with my air-blower. Having stated 'the teeth', I am reminded of three patients who were in a different category. Whereas most patients asked me to check their teeth, three patients would request that I checked their tooth. Yes - they had one tooth each.

The dental examination under the National Health Service was free for the patient, and the dentist received a fixed fee, regardless of how many teeth were present. The patient was pleased that their one tooth was the focus of my attention, and that if any problems arose, I would be sure to find and resolve them. Me? - I was happy to receive a full examination fee for examining one tooth. Then two of the three patients died, and I was left with one. After that, the government decided that patients should pay for their dental examination, and my remaining one-toothed patient told me, apologetically, that he was not going to pay a full examination fee to have one tooth checked. Then he too died!

Why dry the teeth? Because your teeth are wet! The mouth is full of saliva, which is constantly being produced by the various salivary glands. Saliva lubricates the mouth, and also lubricates the food when it is swallowed. It contains enzymes that assist digestion, and - it enables you to spit. If you do that sort of thing.

So I would slowly dry each tooth, and spend a few seconds staring at it. Moisture on the tooth surface would reflect light, and thus obscure the underlying surface detail. Small cavities, shadows indicating decay under the surface, minute cracks in fillings, corrosion on the surface, and particularly at the margins, of amalgam fillings, would usually be quite apparent on a dry tooth, but be totally obscured by reflected light on a damp tooth. And also, of course, a sensitive tooth would usually make itself known with the air-blower.

And then I would probe - with the probe! Scratch, scratch, scratch. I would run the finely sharpened point over *every* surface of *every* tooth. And I would ask myself, "Does it stick, click, catch or grate?" A small cavity (stick), an amalgam with the edge fractured (click), an amalgam with an overhanging edge (catch), or corroded filling (grate), would become apparent *only* by probing every surface of every tooth. These findings would be noted, and discussed with the patient. We might well decide to leave things as they were, but we would at least *know* such lesions existed.

And the final clinical examination was of the gums. A blunt *periodontal* probe was used to measure how deep the little pocket between gum and tooth was. I will spare you a detailed explanation, and will simply say that gums often need attention. Scaling and polishing is not unusual, and is of immense benefit, adding years to the life of the teeth, when appropriate.

"Stick your tongue out now," reminds me of a Tommy Cooper joke. But that is what I said, with a "Move it to the right" and "Move it to the left," to check that muscles were not involved in anything sinister. These days I go back to my old practice in Norwich, and my dentist Charles also says, "Stick your tongue out. To the left. To the right!"

So a dental examination involves more than looking round the mouth, or probing round the mouth. And having concluded the 'check-up', I would explain to the patient the state of their teeth, fillings, gums, and appliances (dentures).

"Any questions?" I would ask.

95% said they had no questions. 4% were straightforward. 1% were a challenge.

I would outline treatment by saying that I 'advised', say, 2 extractions, 5 fillings, a false tooth (plastic or metal denture), gum surgery... and so on.

"No thanks mate," was what Bob Horner said to me every time. Such a polite man, and always, "No treatment thanks." Every six months, he would return for his examination, after which he would hear me say, "Still five fillings and an extraction, Bob."

"No thanks mate," he would say. "Thanks a lot. I'll see you in six months."

And after a further year or two, I would say, "I'm afraid it's six fillings and two extractions now. Are you sure you would not like me to put your mouth in order?"

"No thanks mate. I like them as they are. But thanks for checking them. I'll see you in six months." Bob was a nice guy who liked to do things properly, and no doubt had heard that he should have his teeth checked every six months. But when it came to having them treated....

And after many years, I sold the practice to one of my associates, and Charles 'inherited' Bob. I can imagine Charles checking Bob's teeth and saying, "Twelve fillings, five extractions and a denture." And Bob would say, "No thanks mate. I'll see you in six months."

I wonder if he ever had toothache!

* * *

But there is one other routine procedure that dentists use to investigate the health of the teeth and surrounding jawbone. This again reminds me of an incident in the life of 007.

In the film *You Only Live Twice (1967)*, James Bond is in Japan, masquerading as the overseas representative of an export company. He arranges an appointment with Mr. Osato, head of Osato Chemicals, who is suspected of being highly involved in international villainy. Bond faces Osato, who is sitting behind his desk. Everything appears to be normal, but the camera swings round to reveal a concealed screen in Osato's desk. The picture on the screen? - an X-ray of 007, clearly showing a Walther PPK pistol under his left armpit.

* * *

Susan Henderson and her family had been regular patients of mine for a few years. Her husband was a wealthy farmer, who later secretly (but in partnership with the appropriate govern-ment department) pioneered experimentation with GM crops, and found himself on the front page of several national newspapers when saboteurs and protesters invaded his land, causing incredible damage.

"I'll just take a couple of X-rays of your teeth, Mrs. Henderson," I explained. "It's been two years since the last ones were taken. Oops - sorry! My mistake - I can't really take them while you're pregnant," I added with a degree of embarrassment, to the well-spoken lady with a distinct bulge at the front.

Silence. A reddening of the cheeks.

"Actually, Mr. Lawrence," said the patient, now glaring at me, "I am *not* pregnant."

Now it was my turn to feel uncomfortable. Really uncomfortable. I considered how to respond. And then the patient burst out laughing.

"I'm so sorry," she said, almost crying with hilarity. "It's been Christmas, hasn't it, and I have really over-indulged this year. But I'm certainly not pregnant, so go ahead with the X-rays."

X-rays were discovered by Wilhelm Röntgen in 1895. They are electromagnetic waves which penetrate tissue, such as the human body, and cast a shadow on a photographic film. Dense substances, such as bone, cast dense shadows. Dental enamel casts a very dense shadow, and decayed tooth casts a very light shadow.

Within a year of Röntgen's discovery, a Glasgow hospital had developed an X-ray machine and demonstrated a kidney stone, and a penny lodged in a child's throat. Dental X-rays soon followed. The dangers of radiation, however, were not recognised until those involved started suffering burns, losing hair, and sustaining other irreparable tissue changes. Steps were taken to protect both operators and patients. The dose used in dental surgeries today is extremely low, and together with other protective measures, ensures there is no danger to anyone involved. However, when I was in practice, it was deemed advisable to refrain from taking X-rays on ladies who were pregnant.

So what can be seen on an X-ray, technically called a *radiograph*, that cannot be detected clinically with the naked eye and a sharp dental probe? A very tiny hole on the surface of the tooth might be missed with the probe, but the underlying invasion and destruction of the dentine shows as a dark area on an X-ray. However, the areas that are much more commonly affected, and almost impossible to detect clinically, are the points where the teeth touch each other around the arch. These are called *contact points*, and tend to hold sugar in solution against the enamel, resulting in decay. Such lesions usually show up clearly on the little X-rays one has to bite on, called *bitewings*.

Another use of dental X-rays is in the diagnosis of an abscess, where infected material from the tooth's 'nerve' causes bone to shrink away around the tip of the root. Most dentists these days have panoramic X-ray machines, which will show unerupted, and possibly impacted, wisdom teeth. Occasionally, the X-ray would show something quite extraordinary.

"Have you ever been shot?" I asked Keith Plummer, after staring at his X-ray in near disbelief. "With a gun, that is."

"Cor - how do you know that, mate?" Keith stared at me, wide-eyed in amazement. "Walking across a field by a wood, I was, when some blighter fired out of the trees. Got me on the cheek. Glanced off, it did. Left the hell of a mark. He cleared off, of course."

"That wasn't a 'glancing off' mark," I explained. "That was a 'going in' mark."

"No way. That was ten years ago, mate," replied Keith, who was unconvinced until I showed him the panoramic X-ray of his jaws, with a .22 lead pellet firmly embedded in his mandible. I would not want to print his exclamation of surprise!

So Keith was referred to our local hospital, and although it had given him no trouble, having lead embedded in one's jaw bone is not exactly conducive to good long-term health. So an appointment was arranged for it to be removed. But Keith failed to attend for the procedure, possibly because it was on the afternoon of 24th December, and he wanted to enjoy his Christmas.

And every once in a while, when I took X-rays of Keith's teeth, he would grin and say, "Still there, is it?"

* * *

Patients usually have small X-rays, to check for cavities, taken around once every two years, but the dentist and his team are in the surgery everyday. To make absolutely sure that the dental personnel do not have any overdose, we stand well away from the machine. When I was first in practice, I would place the camera in position next to the patient and operate it with a long cable, standing in the surgery doorway. Later, at my city practice, an X-ray machine was installed that had a timer. I would position the camera pointing at the patient's cheek, press the button, and leave the surgery. Ten seconds later the machine would 'click' and I would know the radiograph had been taken.

"Just sit still while the camera takes the picture," I explained to Jason Brown, a new patient in his early twenties, wearing the standard jeans and T-shirt of his generation. "I'll press a button and leave the room for a few seconds, and then it will be done."

The X-ray film was in Jason's mouth, and the camera in position. I pressed the button and marched briskly out of the surgery. Turning to look back into the room, I saw - Jason had stepped out of the chair, and was crouching down to stare into the tube from which the X-rays were about to emanate! I leapt back through the doorway, and hit the 'Off' switch.

"What are you doing?" I asked rather brusquely, as Jason stared up at me, clearly startled.

"Just wanted to see 'em come out, mate," he explained casually. Well, of course! Lesson - never assume anything.

Peter, a colleague of mine took an X-ray of an upper canine, or eye tooth, which had been tingling and aching intermittently. The resulting picture showed an extremely dense, almost certainly metal, object directly over the tip of the root. Mystery.

What was the object, and how could it have become lodged over the apex of the root? Peter spent a while just staring at the image before returning to take another look at the patient, when all became clear. Natasha had a metal stud adorning her upper lip, and its image had been superimposed over the tip of the canine's root. Dentures, whether plastic or metal, and studs, rings and bolts through lips and tongue, should always be removed prior to X-rays being taken.

* * *

So we were trained to investigate, identify, and eliminate anything invasive to the dentition. Eliminate? - read on!

Chapter 4

Cocaine - and Shots!

He clenched his fist, and pushed it under my nose, saying "Shoot me in the arm, mate."

* * *

Shots! Rather like 007, I have given thousands, maybe tens of thousands over the years. After my first experience of dental treatment where the foul smelling mask was held securely over my infantile hooter until I passed out, I never had a general anaesthetic at the dentist's again, and injections became my number one 'hate'.

The needles were big, long, and thick. They were sterilised in an antiseptic solution in a jar, not dissimilar to those used for storing spaghetti. In the surgery in Shaftesbury, where I practised for five years immediately after I qualified, they hung in such a jar in front of the patient. Once their eyes alighted on them, they froze and remained riveted on them.

"How many times do you use these needles?" I asked my boss in that Dorset practice. "They must lose their sharpness after a while."

"Until you can no longer get them to penetrate the gum," he said with a wry little smile. "They cost money, you know. Private patients are different, but on the NHS, you just keep using them."

It was a crisis of conscience for me, as I pushed quite hard at times until the needle burst through the gum tissue with a jolt.

I did not want to cost the practice unnecessary expense - but the expressions on some patient's faces were not a pretty sight at times.

The fast drill (in contrast to the engine driven slow one) used burs that were made of diamond chippings fused to a shank of stainless steel. At 500,000 rpm, they made short work of dental enamel. Well, that was true the first time the bur was used, but then it started to get smooth. Maybe the second time would be OK, perhaps the eighth.

"How often do I change the bur for a new one?" I asked the practice owner.

"When you can see your face in it!" was his reply. "Burs cost money. Private patients are different, but on the NHS..."

I was young and naïve, and Reg had a mischievous grin as he spoke. With hindsight, I really do not think he was serious, but sadly for my patients at that time, I took him *very* seriously. Well, he was the boss.

* * *

"I'll have the cocaine please," said the rather smart, besuited gentleman who had just sat in my chair, ready to have a tooth extracted.

Cocaine! It had been used towards the end of the nineteenth century, but was history by the time I was being trained in the early '60s. Cocaine was one of a number of substances employed for pain relief in dentistry over the centuries. Wine had also been used to produce insensibility, and likewise curare, better known as the poison placed on Indians' arrows in the Amazon basin.

Lignocaine hydrochloride was the local anaesthetic most commonly used in the second half of the twentieth century in the UK, having reasonably rapid onset and working time, with few side effects. It was first synthesised in Sweden by two scientists who tested it on rodents and found it to be extremely successful. They were travelling by rail to a conference in 1944, where they were to announce their new anaesthetic. Suddenly they realised that they had not demonstrated that it worked on *humans*. Only rodents. Initial alarm gave way to resourcefulness, and the two men proceeded to the toilet, only to reappear a few minutes later with one holding a syringe and the other holding his lower lip. He was still numb when they entered the conference centre.

However, general anaesthetics, including wine and other alcoholic beverages, had been widely used for decades – in fact, wine and alcoholic beverages for millennia. It was during my years in Shaftesbury that I really learnt how to successfully administer general anaesthetics with nitrous oxide and oxygen ('gas'), augmented with a little halothane – and also some experimental stuff. But I will come to that in the next chapter.

* * *

Shots of local anaesthetic were invariably adequate for all normal dental procedures - fillings, extractions, and gum surgery. However, there were occasions when an injection did not work.

The most common cause of acute dental pain is an abscess. Most abscesses emanate from the infected pulpal tissue ('nerve') of a dead tooth. The abscess then leaks bacteria into the surrounding area, which itself becomes infected, inflamed and tender. An injection into such tissue is often ineffective, or only partially successful. This is one reason antibiotics are usually prescribed to resolve the infection before commencing treatment.

Shots in order to numb upper teeth are nearly always effective, whereas there is a significant failure rate with lower teeth. The reason for this is anatomical. The upper teeth are supplied with a multitude of fine nerves descending through the relatively porous maxilla (upper jaw bone). If local anaesthetic is placed in the vicinity of the tooth that one wants to work on, it will diffuse through the bone, and the whole area goes numb.

The lower jaw is very different. The nerve to the lower teeth is thick, like a piece of string, and enters the mandible (lower jaw bone) at the back of the mouth. It then runs along an enclosed tunnel under the lower teeth, with a filament running up to each tooth. Place local anaesthetic beside a lower tooth, and it will numb only the gum. The lower jaw bone is so hard and dense that the anaesthetic will not soak through it. The answer? - the dentist has to numb the nerve in the tissues at the back of the mouth before it enters the canal. There are potential problems - the dentist is 'working in the dark' obviously unable to see the nerve, and the position of the nerve is a little variable. This can be frustrating for the dentist, and more than a little tiresome for the patient. One way I would attempt to overcome this problem was to penetrate until the tip of the needle was very close to the bone, and then squirt hard. It was neither painful nor uncomfortable, and the anaesthetic would scatter widely and soak through a greater area.

And when the dentist is successful in reaching the nerve to the lower teeth, the patient knows. The nerve runs along the canal under the lower teeth, but a branch emerges through a tiny hole and supplies the lower lip. "My lip has just gone numb on the side where you injected," can be music to the ears of a frustrated dentist.

This difficult injection to numb the lower teeth was immortalised in the film *Dentist In The Chair* (1960) where the student dentist directs his gaze into the back of the mouth where he is intending to reach the nerve. He believes his needle has arrived in the correct position, and enthusiastically pushes the plunger into the syringe, causing the anaesthetic solution to be expelled through the needle. But it is not deposited in the vicinity of the nerve. The camera swings round to show what the dental student cannot see - the needle has penetrated deeply and is sticking out through the side of the patient's neck. A great stream of local anaesthetic shoots from the needle, flies across the clinic and hits another patient on the side of the face. As a fifteen year old prospective dental student, I cannot remembering laughing so much as when watching that sequence of the film.

* * *

I was a student at the local grammar school, studying hard to pass the necessary Advanced Level GCE examinations, when I had a problem with a lower molar. Sandy Pitt-Steele, our local all-singing, all-dancing and much loved dentist, diagnosed a problem that needed some attention with the dreaded drill.

"I'll have to numb your tooth first," said Sandy, and broke into song. Well, that was what Sandy did. As mentioned in a previous chapter, he was the talk of the town for months after he first arrived and set up practice in some rooms behind the school I attended.

"Have you seen his medallion swing?" said one of the chaps in my class. Sandy had a large gold medallion on a chain round his neck, and it swung to and fro across his pink silk shirt as he strode energetically through the town, or gyrated round the surgery, often breaking into song, seemingly oblivious to patients and staff.

"That medallion of his," said an attractive blonde clerk working in the same bank as my father. "It went down the front of my blouse when he leant forward to look at my teeth. I gave a shriek - well, it was all cold and tingly on my, er, well, um, down the front of my blouse. When I shrieked, he jumped back, and it shot out. I got the giggles, and Mr. Pitt-Steele burst into song! I suppose it was quite exciting really - if you know what I mean."

So, back to my aching molar which Sandy decided to numb. I opened my mouth as wide as I could, and he painlessly delivered a shot of local anaesthetic into the tissues behind the teeth.

"Have a rinse Barrie," said Sandy.

But I was unable to grasp the tumbler of pink liquid. There were two tumblers, and in fact, there were two Sandys, and two of everything. I blinked, and blinked again. Blink, blink, blink. Despite blinking, there were still two surgeries, nurses, everything.

"I've got double vision," I explained. Sandy asked if I felt faint, which I did not, and helped me back to the waiting room.

Around fifteen minutes later, the problem had resolved. Neither Sandy, nor anyone else I have asked has had a clear explanation of what happened. But I came across it again later, twice.

Gareth Emrys-Jones was a year below me at the dental school. He was taller, broader, deeper and heavier than most of his fellow students, but an altogether decent chap and a star on the rugby field. Also, he was a patient of mine.

"Sorry. I'll need to go in at the back of the mouth for this one," I said, and Gareth opened wide. All went well, until -

"I can't see properly," stammered Gareth. "Everything's double. I've got double vision. What's happened?"

Double vision? I thought that was something our rugby players were more than used to, having observed them crashing back into the students' hostel in the early hours on Sunday mornings.

"Double vision? I will get a registrar to come and have a look, but it did happen to me once," I explained. And by the time the registrar arrived at the chair, Gareth was almost back to normal.

Some years later in practice in Shaftesbury, having delivered a shot to numb the lower teeth, the patient exclaimed,

"It's my eyes. I can't see properly. Everything is double."

So I reassured him that it's a rare occurrence that soon rights itself again. "It happens to dentists, star rugby players, you - all the best people."

* * *

Finally, one of the incidents I shall never forget was when a man entered the waiting room, went to reception and explained that he had been awake several nights with toothache, and just had, *had*, to have the tooth out. Tom Higgins. Money no object. Just do it.

He was clearly a genuine emergency and was shown into my surgery quite promptly. An upper molar had a large cavity, and was probably beyond redemption.

"Just pull it out," said the man with a somewhat strained

expression, pointing to an upper molar with a large cavity. Clearly the tooth needed extracting, and so I picked up my local anaesthetic syringe.

"No need for that," said Tom Higgins. "It's numb already. The fat man zapped it."

"The fat man zapped it?" I repeated. "I don't understand."

"I went to the dentist that people call 'the fat man'. You must know who I mean. Everybody knows the fat man," continued Tom. I thought that I probably did know who he meant. "Well, he didn't speak to me at all when I entered the surgery. Just pointed to the chair. I think he was having a bad day. Reeked of tobacco. He had trouble getting near enough, I think. So fat! I told him the tooth was aching, and he looked at it and swore. He does, you know. Then - *Bang*, in went the needle, and before I knew it, *Bang*, in it went again. He swore a second time - maybe a third or fourth, in fact - and then he and the nurse walked out. I expect they'd gone for a coffee. I crept to the door, and took a cautious look. There was no sign of them, so I took a deep breath, and ran like hell. I'd heard of you, so here I am. Numb. Just take it out please." So I did.

About that time, a friend of mine at church asked me, "Do you know the dentist called 'the fat man'? I saw him in his new Range Rover the other day. It was like one of those puzzle pictures, because three questions immediately came into my mind. Firstly, how does he get in? Secondly, how does he get out? And thirdly, what happens to the steering wheel?" So I think it must have been quite gross, and I could have added a question or two myself, like, 'How does he get close enough to the teeth?', and 'I wonder what he said when he found that his patient had fled?' I expect he swore again. Licensed to drill? - no thanks! But he could give shots. He could numb teeth!

* * *

And then one day, as I was about to gently numb an upper molar, the patient clenched his fist, and pushed it under my nose, saying "Shoot me in the arm, mate." Of course, I could have injected his arm, but the only effect would have been to anaesthetise that part of his anatomy. Which was not what he wanted. I explained this to the gentleman in the chair, and he leant back, opened his mouth, and was probably amazed at how little he felt when I penetrated his gum.

However, this did alert me to those who were too nervous to even countenance seeing the fat man, or any other dentist. So they came to see me. Why? Because they wanted to be 'out cold'. Let me explain further in the next chapter.

Chapter 5

Out Cold

Her eyes stared upwards, unseeing, and her pupils dilated. As her shallow breathing finally stopped, her complexion changed to blue. She was out cold. She had been asphyxiated.

* * *

I have written earlier of my own first experience of dental treatment, when a black rubber mask was placed over my face while I screamed and struggled against overwhelming odds - and succumbed.

During my childhood, few words would cause one's adrenaline to flow more copiously than 'dentist' and 'gas', though the combination, 'school dentist', probably pipped the other two at the post.

"Have you heard? The school dentist is here," were words that sent shock waves round the primary school at Wroxham. It was the mid-1950s, and the staff would keep very quiet about the arrival of this man of torture. But word soon got round, and everybody knew. It must have been similar when the executioner arrived at a prison, where the news would circulate, and everybody would know. In such situations, in both institutions, a deathly hush would descend, and the inmates would quietly whisper to one another.

"They've called Mrs. Shreeve's class through to see him. One at a time. And some haven't come out again," said Sylvia glumly.

"They can't do that. They're not allowed unless your parents have given permission. And *mine* haven't," volunteered Mike.

"Well they're taking them *all* through, one at a time. Whether there's permission or not. And some haven't come back," said Sylvia, this time with a hint of menace in her voice.

Silence descended again upon the little groups in the playground, who would normally have been playing tag, which for some reason was called 'It' at our school, often with a silent 't'. I', as in li"le, bu"er, and li"er. We should really have known be"er.

"Have you heard?" said John, his complexion ashen. "Humbo's been carried out on a stretcher. He's out cold, but still alive. So someone said."

No-one knew how Humbo got his name, or why. Or Gully, or Shadley, or Digger, or Bog Rat. I was later known as Snowball - I had fairly tight, blond curls, and once the first person had called me Snowball, everybody called me Snowball.

"And I've heard that Humbo's parents did *not* give permission," said Sylvia.

"I expect they gave him gas," stuttered Dave. "They're always carried out on stretchers when they've been gassed."

In fact, our class was not called through to see the dentist, and Humbo had *not* been gassed. He had passed out when he was called through, and removed on a stretcher for that reason. The dentist was just examining the teeth of the pupils in the classes of the youngest children, and then the parents were informed of necessary treatment.

Having said that, gas was used extensively where extractions were required in infants and young children. It was feared by most prospective patients, but enjoyed by some members of the dental profession - sadists and addicts.

I suspect that there is a liberal sprinkling of those with sadistic tendencies in most walks of life. One reads accounts of horrendous beatings in schools, of dreadful punishments in the military, and I would be surprised if the dental profession did not have its fair share of cruelly perverse practitioners. However, there were also those who enjoyed the experience of inhaling nitrous oxide themselves.

Addiction. I wonder how an individual ever got started on the inhalation, or 'sniffing', of nitrous oxide. But so many did, and also on stronger substances, such as pethidine. Whilst training during the 1960s, I read of one incident related by a witness giving evidence to the disciplinary committee of the General Dental Council, where a dentist was accused of being unfit to practice due to his addiction to nitrous oxide. According to the national newspaper where I read the story, Mrs. Bloggins (I cannot remember her actual name) had brought young Joey (or Tom or Fred) to the dentist, who had told her to make an appointment for him to have a few painful teeth removed 'under a general anaesthetic'. Gas. *Laughing* gas. Mrs. Bloggins had duly arrived for the extractions appointment, and was shown into the surgery by a nurse. The dentist was not there, and the nurse gave a sigh and walked back out through the door. No sooner had she done so than another door opened, and the dentist entered. He was smiling. Seeing the child in the chair and the mother standing beside him, he stopped. And then he started laughing. Did you ever see those seaside amusements where you inserted a coin and the effigy of a policeman started to laugh? They were called laughing policemen. The newspaper reported that the dentist was just like that. He laughed and he laughed. Then he sat on the floor and laughed some more, after which he tried to stand up, but fell down again. And laughed. Needless to say, he was struck off. Struck off? - indefinitely suspended from practising dentistry unless and until he could persuade the committee that he was no longer addicted to the practice of sniffing the nitrous oxide gas.

The above story was not uncommon in those days, but the one I have related had a scary footnote. The dentist who was struck off was around sixty years of age, and did not want to lose his practice. The solution? His mother, aged ninety, being a qualified, though retired dentist herself, stepped in and took over the practice until her son returned. Ninety? Some people would rather be treated by an addict.

Reflecting on our training at dental school, we had little experience of administering general anaesthetics. I recall observing two or three gas sessions, and I never saw a patient anaesthetised intravenously (needle-in-the-arm). One memorable incident at dental school involved a patient coming in for an extraction with a *local* anaesthetic – and ending up 'out cold'.

A new senior registrar in oral surgery had most of the staff talking. His appearance was part-Neanderthal and part-gorilla, with a chair-side manner to match. It went well with his heavy South African accent. A local man, with a nervous disposition and a badly decayed tooth that had been keeping him awake at night, had eventually decided that even a visit to the dentist would be preferable to continued pain from the tooth. Until he caught sight of the new registrar. Walking in to the clinic where the Neanderthal-Gorilla was standing beside the dental chair, he stopped dead in his tracks. His eyes rolled up and he collapsed in a heap. Out cold! Without a second's hesitation, and in front of around a dozen wide-eyed, almost disbelieving dental students, King Kong grabbed the forceps, knelt beside the patient, and removed the tooth with a mighty jerk. The patient was no longer 'out cold', and giving a shout, leapt to his feet and was led to a recovery room by a rather startled nurse.

The huge unkempt shaggy creature turned to us with a wry grin. "Seize the moment. The tooth is out, the patient has been brought round from their faint, and all without having to give an injection." Today there would be disciplinary hearings, suspension, litigation......

* * *

I qualified in December 1968, and in my absence, was likened to a monkey with a pistol being let loose on the population – those memorable words spoken by the unforgettable Dudley

Farmer, Senior Registrar and lecturer in Dental Surgery at the London Hospital.

The monkey drove down to Shaftesbury in Dorset, where Reg Carnall had decided that Barrie Lawrence was *not* a monkey with a pistol, but a colleague with a future. I will always be grateful to Reg, and it was there at his practice in the house named *Rockcliffe* that I first administered general anaesthetics using nitrous oxide, oxygen and a small amount of halothane to give it potency.

Reg showed me how to check the oxygen level, and attach the cylinders to the machine. The halothane was extremely expensive, and used sparingly. One sniff could knock you out, but the stream of nitrous oxide and oxygen passed over the halothane, which vaporized and was carried along in small quantities. Children went to sleep quickly, and we preferred adults to have treatment carried out under a local anaesthetic. But not everyone was willing.

"We have a gypsy coming in for an extraction today," said Reg. "It's your turn to give the G.A., which could prove to be something of a challenge. And I will carry out the extraction, which could be another challenge."

The words 'general anaesthetic' were something of a mouthful (if you will excuse the pun), and so we used to say 'G.A.'. It sounded more professional than "We're going to gas a gypsy today."

He was a large muscular man in early middle-age. He strode into the surgery, and sat in our cast-iron dental chair as though he was settling down for an evening's television.

We placed one heavy duty strap over his knees to keep his legs and feet down, and another round his chest to prevent him lurching forwards and leaving the chair. I placed the mask over his nose and mouth, and he breathed deeply. His eyes closed and his face started going even redder than when he had entered the room. And then he reached the excitability stage.

We were taught that there are various stages that a patient passes through before becoming totally anaesthetised, and the excitability stage was the one we hoped they would pass through quickly. Indeed, it hardly occurred at all with some people. The gypsy however, was different, as he started rocking backwards and forwards. Then the cast iron chair started rocking with him. I was standing behind the patient, holding the mask over his face and trying to hang onto him as the chair rocked backwards and forwards, advancing each time by a few inches across the surgery towards Reg, who was trying to extract the tooth whilst walking backwards to prevent being assaulted by the chair bearing down on him. Somehow, we all survived the experience, but this was one reason that caused me to consider alternative ways that would be less traumatic for both patient and dentist.

Most doctors and dentists involved in the administration of G.A.s had stories to tell. On a course in Exeter on the subject of general anaesthetics, a doctor in general practice told me that his local dentist often asked him to come and give the 'gas' when one of his patients wanted a tooth out that way. On one occasion the patient was sitting in the chair, the doctor had the mask in place, while the dentist patiently waited on the far side of the surgery. After a couple of minutes or so, the patient's eyes rolled up, and then his eyelids closed. He was breathing regularly, and the doctor waited a further minute or so before looking across at the dentist, nodding towards the forceps, and saying "OK?"

"I'm fine thanks!" said the patient with his eyes still closed, to the surprise of both doctor and dentist. Those were strange days!

* * *

Bill Roberts (not his real name) came to work at my first practice in the city of Norwich. He was keen to be a successful dental surgeon, had a great sense of humour, was a practising Christian, and proved to be a complete scatterbrain.

"Can I give the G.A. today?" asked Bill, seeing that we had two or three children coming in for extractions under a general anaesthetic.

He had administered several already, and was really struggling to master the technique. He was a warm, caring young man, but you would not have guessed that from his manner at times. There was a hint of impatience in the way he was economic with words. "Come in", "Open your mouth", "Wider, wider!" were barked out with a total absence of 'Please" or 'Thank you." I spoke to him about it, and he said he would try harder, but he was not a great listener either.

A lady with her five year old daughter entered the surgery.

"Good morning, Mrs. Dellow," I greeted the mother, and "Hello Lucy. What is the name of the dolly you are hugging?" I enquired.

"Sit down," came from the other end of the surgery, and I held Lucy's hand and helped her into the chair.

"Breathe," said Bill, as I continued to hold Lucy's hand and smile at her. Lucy looked apprehensive, but her mother gave her a nervous smile, and, as Lucy's eyes closed, she left the surgery. I turned to have another look at the records. Where extractions are being carried out, double and treble checking the teeth to be removed was standard practice for me.

I turned back to the patient. Bill was staring through the end wall of the surgery, probably trying to decide what he wanted for his supper that evening. But Lucy was going blue.

"Bill," I said very sternly, "Your patient is turning blue. What's happening?"

Her eyes stared upwards, unseeing, and her pupils dilated. As her shallow breathing finally stopped, her complexion changed to blue. She was out cold.

Bill looked down at his patient, and went as white as a sheet – then panicked. 'Blue," he stammered, staring down at her. "Blue," he blurted out, and stood there staring at Lucy, who seemed to have stopped breathing.

I physically pushed him well clear of the patient so that I had full access. Pulling the mask away, I pressed my index finger very firmly over the carotid artery in the right side of her neck. I suspect that the pressure from my finger caused pain, because

Lucy jerked forwards and gave a great gasp – and started breathing again. I quickly removed the offending tooth, and gave the patient some light slaps to bring her round quickly. All was well, and mother and daughter left the practice with a smile.

But I was not smiling, and nor was Bill. What had happened, and why? Bill sat slumped across his desk in the corner of the room, and I quickly inspected the gas machine. Scatterbrained Bill had not checked the oxygen cylinders, and had fitted two empty ones. His patient had certainly been 'out cold'; not anaesthetised, but asphyxiated. He vowed he would never give a general anaesthetic again.

* * *

There were other problems with general anaesthetics in general dental practice. One of the first things I did at my Norwich practice, was to transform the two dental chairs I had inherited with the premises. I could not afford the new low-level chairs, but had low-level tops fitted to the existing cast-iron bases. Dentists were at that time being encouraged to work sitting down, whereas it had previously been a standing profession. I had heard that 90% of dentists had back problems later in life, and that 50% had varicose veins. Before too many years had passed, nearly all dentists were sitting to work – and developing neck problems instead. One chap who trained with me had such serious neck problems that he had to retire whilst still a relatively young man.

But the low level chairs undoubtedly saved the lives of at least a few patients, and the IQs of several more. Occasionally a patient would die under a dental general anaesthetic, for no known reason. Others might overhear relations saying, "Uncle Charlie was never the same after he had his teeth out." Indeed, Uncle Charlie may well have changed forever, as eventually became clear. Many of the unexplained deaths, and largely of children, were due to the patient fainting whilst under the anaesthetic. Fainting occurs when the blood drains from the head into the lower parts of the body, due to nervous factors. The person then falls to the ground, and the blood flows back to the brain. An undetected faint during a dental anaesthetic administered with the patient sitting in an upright chair resulted in the brain being starved of oxygen, and the patient liable to sustain damage resulting in impaired mental faculties, or even death. As low-level tops were fitted to both chairs in my Norwich practice, general anaesthetics were always administered safely. Unless Bill Roberts was around.

* * *

When seeking financial backing for the Norwich practice, I was warned not to even consider buying it by those institutions that *always* lent money to dentists. They told me I was the exception that proved the rule, and would not lend me a penny, describing the practice as a 'dead duck'. But I found a bank that would lend me the money as a ten-year loan, and my wife and I prayed that the number of patients would be greater than my predecessor had entertained. He had seen a maximum of eight patients a day, four days a week. I opened in January 1974, and was inundated with patients. The loan was paid off in ten months, and the second surgery, which was sparsely furnished, hardly equipped, and used solely for taking denture impressions, was reburbished, and I took on my first associate dentist a year after starting. But before long I had five surgeries in the premises, and dental surgeons and patients, nurses, hygienists, receptionists and secretaries scurrying around. The relevance of this was that there was a lot of demand for general anaesthetics, and I decided that I would be the one to administer them.

Most of the patients for G.A.s were children, and I remembered my own experience at Mr. Matthew's surgery every time a child walked in. I would jokingly tell my friends that "I love gassing little children", but the truth was that I had found a way that took them through the appointment without distress. I would smile. I would squat down to their level, and talk to them. I would ask about toys, and what their favourite food was, and so on and so forth. I would stand behind the child and stroke their forehead with my left thumb, holding the mask at around waist height. The nitrous oxide would waft around the child while we talked about toys and suchlike, and they would become quite drowsy. I would slowly bring the mask up to their face, and they would generally be as good as asleep by the time I placed it over their nose and mouth. There were minor problems involved, one being that it took time and it took gas, and generally being conducted under the National Health Service, I made a significant financial loss every time I carried out this treatment. But that was insignificant when compared with the satisfaction of seeing a child fall asleep with a smile, and then wake up again with a smile. The second problem? With so much gas wafting around, I wondered if there was a danger of me and/or the nurse falling asleep before the patient! But that never happened.

However, the days of using gas were coming to an end, and I had already started using a totally different method. As I have related in an earlier chapter, it was during my first five years in practice, while I was in Shaftesbury, that I considered the possibility of using a 'needle in the arm' technique. And having experimented to some extent there, I undertook further training whilst in Norwich, and 'shots' in the arm became a normal part of surgery life. Initially they were to leave the patient 'out cold', but later it was sufficient to give a heavy sedation.

* * *

Dentists gave injections in the mouth, and gassed some patients. But back in Shaftesbury, I was occasionally asked if I could do 'the needle in the arm job'. I suspect that the patients asking this read the *Daily Mail*. (If you have a phobia of dental treatment, *do not* read the *Daily Mail*. Dead teeth cause heart attacks and strokes, as do root filled teeth. So have them extracted. And Indian curries cause gum disease....)

'The needle in the arm job' referred to intravenous general anaesthesia. Usually, a barbiturate was injected into a vein in the arm, or the back of the hand, and well within fifteen seconds, the patient was 'out cold'. There was clearly some demand for this procedure, which no other dentist in our area was carrying out, to my knowledge. I met Dick Wilson, an enthusiastic young doctor, new to the town, and we planned our attack.

A fortnight or so later, our first 'IV patient' arrived. IV? – *intravenous*, indicating that it was a procedure where one entered a vein. He was medically fit, had eaten nothing for twenty-four hours, and was accompanied by a friend. Dick shot him in the arm and he was almost immediately out cold. I inserted a pad to protect the throat, a prop to keep the mouth open, and used the forceps to remove the tooth. The patient was soon coming round, though quite disorientated. With such cases we had the chaperone bring their car, or a pre-arranged taxi, to the gate at the end of the garden path leading to the front door. Then Dick would take them by the armpits, and I would take their ankles, or *vice versa*, and we would run along the path to the gate with the patient, and lay them on the back seat of the vehicle. There was a small but steady demand for this, and word got round the town about when these sessions were taking place – resulting in a small crowd assembling on the pavement opposite the practice, to watch the victims being carried out to the waiting vehicles. Before long, Reg, whose practice it was, understandably asked me to discontinue. But later I had my own practice.

* * *

From the outset, the Norwich practice was extremely busy, and for my first few years, I never considered embarking on IV procedures. But adding surgeries and taking on additional dentists enabled me to stand back and consider the needs of the community we were serving. I was especially aware of nervous patients who had a phobia of 'needles in the mouth' and yet who enquired about 'needles in the arm'. I joined a dental society that specialised in anaesthetics, and did further training at

a London hospital, before embarking on intravenous anaesthetics. I gave the anaesthetic, and one of my associates would
carry out the treatment. When the patient started twitching, I
gave them another little shot, and so on until the treatment was
complete. Legally, there had to be two qualified dentists, or
doctor and dentist, present. One problem was that my young
associate dentists were so slow, in a situation where speed was
of the essence. The answer was that I would administer the
anaesthetic whilst my associate stood with the drill at the ready.
The patient would rapidly become unconscious, at which point
I would grab the drill and prepare the teeth for treatment. My
associate would then become the anaesthetist and monitor the
pulse, etc. If the patient started twitching, I would hand the
drill to the associate, and become the anaesthetist again, giving
a small further shot of barbiturate. Then a further exchange of
rôles, and so on.

Patients reacted in different ways after such an anaesthetic.
There were some memorable incidents, including a lady patient
being taken home in the back of her boyfriend's open-top
sports car. She laughed hilariously all the way (maybe a mile)
to the end of the road, her manic cackles reverberating off the
buildings lining the street for several minutes.

Another lady became quite animated as she emerged from a
heavy sedation. "You should see me at parties, darling. I am
wild! Absolutely wild. You should see me - and you must. Fun,
darling. I am *fun!* Just take me to a party....." I made sure I was
never, ever, left alone in the surgery with a patient during *any*
treatment session.

Another patient was entrusted to his chaperone, with the
instruction, "Sit with him while he recovers, because his
judgement will be impaired for up to twenty-four hours. I will
come and check him in twenty minutes." A few minutes later,
we heard brakes screeching outside the practice, and from the
first-floor staff room, I saw a drunken figure lurching across the
road, whilst cars and trucks braked sharply, blew their horns,
and wove around him. I virtually fell down the stairs, dashed

out through the front door and pulled him back into the waiting room.

"What do you think is going on?" I said to his wife, who had her purse open at the reception hatchway. "He's alright dear," she explained calmly. "He's often like that when he comes home from the pub Friday night, and can cope quite well. He was going to the fish and chip shop over the road because he was hungry. Nothing wrong with my Fred."

I learnt a few things that I was not taught on courses too. A huge lady came in for an IV. She had arms like enormous turnips hanging from her shoulders, and the veins were obscured under pounds of fat. As I repeatedly stabbed her arms, hoping I might strike blood, she just laughed at me. Eventually we filled the staff room sink with hot water and left her with both arms submerged for twenty minutes. It worked - but not at subsequent appointments, and I eventually abandoned trying and referred her to the local hospital.

We had no emergencies and generally, patients really appreciated the IV facility. But elsewhere in the UK this was not the case, and in one region especially, there were fatalities under IV general anaesthetics. Questions were asked in parliament, and more and more legislation was introduced. I did more and more courses, and obtained more and more expensive equipment. Then dentists were banned from giving general anaesthetics, and we gave heavy sedations instead. More and more legislation was passed, and I went on more and more courses, and bought more and more expensive equipment. When I retired, I felt a degree of relief, stifled by bureaucracy and legislation concerning, not just anaesthesia and sedations, but small electric appliances such as heaters, plugs for wash-basins, and toilet cleaning liquids.

* * *

I also did some training in another form of 'anaesthesia', though some of my Christian friends would not approve. Hypnosis, to some people, conjures up pictures of people on a stage being put into weird trances by an entertainer, who causes them to quack, bark, and act like idiots. There is a suggestion that hypnosis leaves one vulnerable to sinister spiritual forces. Now, I have no doubt that these powers of darkness exist, and operate in people's lives, causing great harm and distress. We read about them in the Bible, especially but not exclusively, in the New Testament. Another Christian told me he felt that if medical hypnosis left us vulnerable, how much more must be the case while we sleep. But this is a much bigger subject than can be discussed here.

Hypnosis - the word is derived from the Greek word *hypnos*, which means *sleep*. I went on a course at Cambridge University, and my understanding of what I was taught is that we induced relaxation in our patients. We would ask them to daydream about something that appealed to them, perhaps being at a football match or a concert or similar. "Imagine you are walking along Carrow Road to Norwich City Football Ground. You are passing through the turn-stiles, and - Hey, the teams are coming out. What colours do you see?" And so the patter continued.

On the residential course at Churchill College in Cambridge, there was an interesting experience. The lecturer was going through the patter, and then told us to break for coffee. We trooped off - but then realised we were one short. Lee Wong was still sitting on his chair gazing vacantly out into space.

I used the technique on occasions over a two or three year period, during which there were one or two memorable moments. On one occasion when using the football patter, the young man in the chair reached up and pulled my hand away from his mouth and said, "Hey mate. There's been a goal. You should have seen it. The ball came off the crossbar, came back and hit the b*gger on the head, and went into the net." On another occasion the lady who had been enduring the patter for around ten minutes, said, "Oh, just shut up, and give me an injection." On another, the nurse slipped off her stool!

But it took time. It was unpredictable, as some people were

far more susceptible than others. Also, I did not know how to charge for it.

However, from a spiritual perspective, I was confident that most of my patients were not being left vulnerable to dark spiritual forces. Most of my patients were not born-again Christians, and so were open to such forces 24/7 anyway. Patients who were Christians, and therefore members of the family of God, were protected by him. Well, what sort of Heavenly Father do *you* think we have?

Cocaine, shots and 'out cold' are all words and expressions that are used in connection with those who are 'licensed to drill'. Interestingly, so is the word *kill*. I shall explain a little more about killing in the next chapter.

Chapter 6

To Russia with Love

There were three of them. Russians. Two stood and observed coolly as the third carried out the hit. I could only stand and watch, unable to prevent the killing. Death was almost instantaneous.

* * *

The above account is not a scene from the film *From Russia with Love (1963)*. I was actually there, and I saw it. It was Moscow, the winter of February 1987. The temperature was sub-zero day after day, and we lived on *borsht*, the thinnest of cabbage soups with small slithers of animal fat occasionally floating to the surface, doing a circuit, and submerging again.

"Please don't leave any of the vegetables," pleaded Peter. "They will only serve them up again tomorrow. There's a small potato that's been served for three nights running now. I put a secret mark on it, you see. So I know."

As we left the hotel restaurant - or was it a dining-hall, or refectory? - the waiters emerged from the shadows where they had been hiding, waiting for us.

"Caviar? Cheap. Very cheap. English money please. Very cheap."

I was on a dental study tour of the Soviet Union, and we had been taken round the Dental Institute in Moscow. Patients seemed to be kept waiting for hours while the dentists sat around in the clinical areas reading magazines and laughing together. Occasionally a short sturdy lady, built like a Russian tank, would stride to the waiting area and bark out a name such as 'Petrov'.

"*Petrov!*" The sound reverberated around the clinic, echoing down stone corridors as a shabbily dressed pudding-like man slowly got up from his chair and meekly followed the 'nurse' to an upright cast-iron chair. The equipment could have been stolen from the British Museum. A large stainless steel syringe with a needle which, I suspected, had been used so many times that it was blunt, was being leant on by a skinny student in a white, very creased, soiled clinical coat. Maybe he had slept in it. Eventually the needle penetrated the gum, the student lurched forward, but Mr. Pudding did not even blink.

Together with two Russian dental students from the Institute, we were called over to observe a procedure. An air-turbine (sometimes called 'the fast drill' by patients) was produced and almost creaked as it gained speed, at last becoming a shrill whistle. The patient opened his mouth, and the student treating him started pushing the diamond tipped drill onto the tooth surface. My colleagues and I blinked, took a second look, and stared at each other. The drill should have had a copious jet of water playing onto the tooth surface to prevent overheating - but we could see that it was not even plumbed in. There was an arc of red-hot tooth tissue about two millimetres from the point being drilled, and a distinct smell of burning. The tooth may have been anaesthetised, but the live pulpal tissue, or 'nerve', would have died instantly. He had killed his patient's tooth – instant death. And there was nothing we could do but watch. Death was almost instantaneous. I kept my mouth shut.

* * *

It was my first, and last, study tour of dentistry in a foreign country. They were quite popular at the time as those taking part not only toured dental institutes and clinics, but also enjoyed numerous excursions to sites of interest - and restaurants. And it could all be claimed against tax.

I had been to a briefing meeting early in January that year. There had been heavy snow in East Anglia, and my wife and I had been marooned in our cottage. But we had a good stock of curry powder, red wine and James Bond videos, and found the experience exciting. Philip Norton, the farmer who lived a little further along the lane, arrived each day on his tractor bringing eggs and milk. Every lunch time we joined our neighbours, Bob who managed an oil rig and could not get there, and his wife Lynn, a local doctor who was unable to reach her practice. They walked along the top of the hedge on the left side of the road, and we walked along the top of the hedge on the right. We snowballed each other all the way to the pub, downed a pint of beer, and snowballed each other all the way back again.

On the third day I dug my wife's front-wheel drive car out of the snow, and we reached Norwich station and caught the train to London. The briefing meeting was fascinating. Apart from the fact that we were all dentists, and dentists' wives, we were a mixed bunch. All ages, all sizes, some newly qualified, and one a consultant oral surgeon. And all relishing a tax efficient holiday. Sorry, I mean 'study tour'.

"Be prepared for anything," said the briefing officer. "The Soviet Union is notorious for shortages, and not just food. Six months ago there was a dearth of toilet seats in the country, and we advised people to take their own. The entire party was taken to one side at Moscow airport and told to open their suitcases for a search. And there, on top of all their clothes, was a toilet seat. Every one. A row of around thirty. What a photo opportunity! Except you are not allowed to take photographs at Moscow airport."

There were other instructions.

"Russians love children, so do take photographs of your children. And enamel badges - they love them. Also just now, there is a national shortage of contraceptives, so take a good supply because you can exchange them for almost anything. Enamel badges and contraceptives - as many as you can manage, and trade them for caviar."

"Clothes. They are not good quality, and if you can show them a label with 'Marks and Sparks' on it, or any British label, you can trade. But do so in the open, in daylight, and in company. One poor blighter on our last trip arranged to meet some locals after dark in a back street near the hotel. He was found unconscious, and naked. Even his under pants had gone. Maybe they were Marks and Sparks! Be careful when you're there."

We flew to Moscow with Aeroflot, and arrived to find the city enshrouded in snow. Ladies built like battleships were out in the streets with shovels. 'Zhanna, stevedore in the docks, mother of twenty-six, snow-shoveler, and Hero of the Soviet Union' came to mind. I kept my mouth shut.

We were taken on tours of clinics and surgeries and dental schools. We gazed in disbelief as teeth glowed with red heat, and were marched swiftly past a patient who had passed out and was slumped across the arm of the chair. I kept my mouth shut.

A plain clothes gentleman in an MI5-type mackintosh was clearly trailing us as we toured the city, browsing the counters of the mega-store GUM where foreigners and well-heeled, well-dressed Russians were paying for their purchases in dollars. "Vee only accept the dollars here you know. Plees - dollars. Dollars plees." We explored the Kremlin, where permitted, and crossed Red Square to enter Saint Basil's Russian Orthodox Church. Our man from the KGB duly followed us.

Mark was something of a comedian, and gave some of us a nudge and a wink as he broke free and walked up to the KGB man. "Thought you might be interested, comrade," said Mark smiling at Nikita, who was about three feet from him and seemed to be totally oblivious to the fact that he was being addressed. "We plan on being around an hour in here, so you might like to go and have a coffee. Cheers!"

We sauntered into Saint Basil's, still followed by our faithful KGB tail. I kept my mouth shut.

We were taken to a workers' club, where the young people were excited and anticipating almost instant Western standards, goods, culture and general level of living, now that Gorbachev was president. They were to be disappointed of course, but for now were more than satisfied as they filled their pockets with enamel badges and contraceptives. Mark had done his homework, but seemed unsure how to exchange the huge wads of roubles that had been thrust upon him. I kept my mouth shut.

We travelled from Moscow to Leningrad (now Saint Petersburg, its pre-Stalin name) on a steam train called the Red Arrow. It was posh, with a smartly uniformed guard bringing coffee, in an exquisite coffee service, to each sleeper. But it was not so posh when we found that the toilet was blocked, and that a hole had been drilled in the floor instead. Interesting. We were glad to be young and agile.

We slept four to a carriage, separated by curtains. The other dentist and his wife were from the north of England. We introduced ourselves, and passed the time of night. I mentioned that I was an evangelical Christian of the born-again variety. At this, John leapt off his bunk, threw open the door and screamed down the corridor, "Help! I've got an evangelist in my carriage." I think it was the vodka.

In Leningrad we visited Dental Clinic Number 327 - well, something like that - and the director showed us a state-of-the-art laser. We had not seen one before, and the director had no idea how to use it. There had been an exhibition of dental equipment in the city, and one company was able to promote itself back in the USA with words including, 'and donated a dental laser to the people of Leningrad attending clinic number 327.' It saved the expense of shipping it back across the Atlantic. Or perhaps the Pacific.

We walked across the frozen River Neva, explored the Hermitage Museum, and had ice-cream on Gorky Avenue. Our flight home with Aeroflot was scheduled to be direct, but a Russian colonel on board pulled rank on the captain and we landed in Copenhagen to let the gentleman disembark before proceeding to Heathrow.

"Your practice accounts," said my accountant with a somewhat puzzled expression. "One sheepskin coat with matching hat and gloves, used exclusively in the pursuit of your profession? Can you explain that to me please?" In fact, the use of the sheepskin clothes was almost exclusively confined to the time in the Soviet Union. We rarely have weather like that in the East of England, and with all the bread, potatoes, puddings, cakes, and yet more potatoes, few of us ever wore those clothes again after the Russian winter of 1987.

* * *

Death. Teeth die every day for a variety of reasons. The usual reason is simple dental decay. Every time we eat sugar, which is a component of such a wide variety of foods, from the obvious, such as confectionery, to the less likely such as cans of baked beans, sugar remains on the tooth surface. Over the course of twenty minutes or so, it breaks down to form an acid, which dissolves some of the calcium from the enamel, resulting in it eventually becoming porous. Bacteria penetrate to the softer, more vulnerable dentine and infect and destroy it. When they reach the live pulpal tissue, or nerve, it dies. The tooth is now dead. The infected dead pulp often causes an abscess, which is defined as 'a localised collection of pus' just under the tip of the root. Acute pain suggests the tooth is alive, but it is in fact a dead tooth sitting in acutely inflamed, infected bone and gum. A root canal treatment or extraction is indicated.

Another cause of tooth death is trauma. Falling on one's face, or sustaining a blow to the mouth, can both result in the pulpal tissue dying. The blow causes the little blood vessels entering the tooth through tiny holes in the tip of the root, to rupture. As oxygen is no longer being carried into the tooth, it dies. Sooner or later, an abscess usually develops.

* * *

But over the nearly forty years that I was in practice, a large proportion of the real killers went undetected. They smiled and said, "Nice to see you, Mr. Smith," or "Now, how can I help you today?" Some of them were nice guys, and some of the female variety. It was reported to me that many of them hardly said a word, but simply proceeded to... kill.

You have probably guessed the identity of these hidden killers. They were dentists. The deaths of thousands of teeth were unintentional, and took place for many years without anyone being aware that it was happening.

In the early days of 'modern dentistry' - the years when treatment was carried out by trained dental surgeons as opposed to blacksmiths and barbers - the toxic nature of some materials used to restore teeth was not realised. Amalgam, which has been used by the mega-ton over the decades, is approximately fifty percent mercury, which is extremely toxic, though largely inert when chemically alloyed to the silver and tin that comprise most of the remaining fifty percent. But the story gets worse.

Until the mercury has combined chemically with the silver and tin, it is dangerous. This was not understood, and the dental nurse used to mix the materials in her bare hands. Mercury can be absorbed through the skin, entering the small blood vessels there and is eventually deposited in the kidneys. There were many recorded cases of nurses developing renal failure in their fifties, and I have seen sections through the kidneys of some who died from mercury poisoning. Later, it was mixed in a protective rubber, condom-shaped appliance. Today, if amalgam is used, it is bought in airtight capsules, which are vigorously shaken in a machine that achieves near-perfect mixing of the constituents. The nurse and dentist wear rubber gloves and masks, and a high-powered suction unit is in close proximity to the amalgam as it is inserted into the cavity.

Safe? Maybe not. There is still a hidden and invisible killer associated with dental amalgam. Vapour. Viewed under some forms of lighting, mercury vapour can be seen billowing from the liquid material. This can be inhaled, and enters the blood stream through the lungs, lodging in various parts of the body. The nuns in a convent on the continent have generously volunteered to have their memory and co-ordination monitored during their lifetimes, and these readings are correlated to the number of amalgam fillings and the amount of mercury found in their brains at post-mortem.

Today, amalgam fillings are thought to be safe, though increasingly, other mercury-free materials are used to restore teeth. I have many amalgam fillings in my mouth, and it does not bother me one iota. But then, maybe my brain is no longer functioning properly! I jokingly tell people that I do not get dental decay anymore – just rust!

However many people, mainly members of the profession, have died as a result of mercury poisoning, and the number of teeth that have been seen off is far greater. In the early days of 'fillings', the amalgam would be placed into the cavity without placing a protective lining first. Not only would hot and cold drinks sometimes cause extreme sensitivity, but the live 'nerve' would be inflamed by these temperature change shocks, in addition to the close proximity of the villainous mercury.

So linings were introduced. They were cements based on inert substances such as silica, as were some of the tooth-coloured filling materials for front teeth. But they were mixed with an acid to make them set. 'Ouch' - if a dental nerve could speak. Some curled up and quietly died, giving no signs or symptoms. Later, the dead pulpal tissue (nerve) was invaded by bacteria, and not having the defensive cells that blood carries to live parts of the body, developed an abscess. "Oh dear, I am sorry to say that your tooth needs either a root treatment or an extraction."

But everything has moved on from those days, and lining materials tend to soothe rather than irritate. There are stringent regulations regarding all materials used by dentists. Over the past few decades there have been huge advances in all aspects of dentistry, and everyone involved, from dental nurses to patients, and the nerves in their teeth, are quite secure in a twenty-first century dental surgery in the UK.

Russia? I can still see the three Russians, where one attacked the tooth with a waterless high-speed drill while the other two dental students watched it die. However, we were told that this was a dramatic improvement on the dental treatment carried out in the days when Stalin presided over the State, and much of the population was terrified of the KGB, the secret police. The story continued that as so many people were too afraid to open their mouths, dentists had to develop an anal approach - and imagine the damage that could cause. Well, so the joke goes.

But I'm keeping my mouth shut.

Chapter 7

Goldentooth

Goldeneye was the Bond film released in 1995. I watched it many times. The plot was just about OK, and Pierce Brosnan was perhaps my fourth favourite 'James Bond'. Sean Bean and Judi Dench never disappoint, but it was Famke Janssen playing Xenia Onatopp who stole the show for me.

Ian Fleming never wrote a Bond book with the title Goldeneye, but it was the name of the house he lived in on the north coast of Jamaica. There are birds called goldeneyes, though Fleming said the property was named after *Operation Goldeneye*, which he had devised while working with Naval Intelligence during World War ll, in the event of Gibraltar falling to the Nazis through an invasion via Spain.

* * *

"I want this tooth crowned, and I want it in gold," said the rather slick young man in the sharp suit.

I had not even examined his teeth, but he was pointing to a molar, and asking me to crown it. "Gold," he emphasised.

It was heavily filled, but did not need crowning. I explained that the tooth was quite sound, and did not *need* a crown.

"But I want one, and that's what I'm asking you to do. When you do cosmetic crowns for people's front teeth, they don't *need* crowning. It's just what they want. And I'm asking you to crown this back tooth. I don't expect the NHS will want to know, but I'm prepared to pay. How much is a private gold crown?"

I quoted £150, and Max Spellman said that there would be no problem. Maybe the molar *would* need crowning one day, and doing so now might just prevent a filling fracturing in future, which could be painful.

So two appointments were arranged, and I duly crowned Max's molar. He paid cash at reception, and left with a smile.

I did not see Max again in my surgery, but one of my young associates did.

"I've had a really strange experience with a patient you used to see called Max Spellman," said Chris. "There was a molar that you had crowned privately around a year ago, and he wanted me to extract it. I said that he should see you, but he wanted to see me. And he wanted me to make him a false tooth to fill the gap it would leave. But there was nothing wrong with it, as far as I could see. I took X-rays - but nothing. So he continued complaining about the pain, but I think he was pretending. Maybe I was wrong, but I made a denture for him, took the tooth out, and put the false one in. He insisted on having the extracted tooth, and I'm sure he was smiling to himself as he left. A lopsided smile - but a smile."

It was a month or two later that I saw Max walking along the road on which my city practice was situated. I caught his eye, but he was not smiling back at me.

"I've been done," he exclaimed, looking more than indignant. "Why do you charge people £150 for a gold crown?"

I explained that I ran a surgery full of expensive equipment, and had skilled staff who I tried to pay appropriately. Gold was expensive, but I also had to pay the technician who made the crown. He too was highly skilled, and used a laboratory full of expensive equipment.

Max paused and thought. "Well, I wish I'd known all that a year ago," he replied. "I'm not stupid, you know. And I will make money like the big boys do. But I really feel cheated with that crown?"

I asked him what the problem was, and why he had asked Chris to extract the tooth, and not come back to me, if there had been a problem. He said that he did not think I would extract the tooth for him, so he went to a younger dentist.

But why? I felt I was missing something in all this.

"It's the gold, Mr. Lawrence. Gold! I'm not stupid, and one day I'll really make a killing. But I'm learning all the time. I read the *Daily Express*, you see, and they give financial recommendations. Gold. That's what they've been tipping. So I thought I would take advantage of it, and get hold of some gold. So, I came to you for a crown, and then I just watched the price of gold every day. And they were right, and it's gone up and up. So I saw the young dentist at your place, and he took the crowned tooth out for me. On the NHS, and together with a plate, only cost about fifty quid. So I wrapped up my golden tooth and took it to a jeweller in the city. And what did he offer me? Five quid. Just five quid. So I went elsewhere, but they're all the same. £150 that cost me, plus £50 to your mate. And I'm offered five quid. I can't help thinking I've been done."

It was a sad tale, but if someone wants to invest in gold, there are far more efficient ways than having your teeth crowned.

* * *

I loved gold as a material for restoring teeth. It never corroded, and was a warm friendly material to work with.

At dental school, we were taught to fill non-stress bearing areas (the sides of back teeth) with pure gold. 24 carat. Small flakes of gold were hammered into the cavity. The hammering work-hardened the material, and they could last a lifetime.

Gold Inlays were small fillings cast in the laboratory, and cemented into the prepared cavities. They were 18 carat gold, meaning 75% gold. The other 25% was mainly copper. Crowns were made the same way and of the same material, but instead of going in the tooth, they went on and around the tooth. But I will spare you the clinical details, as this is not a clinical book.

* * *

"Have you seen Mrs. Davenport's teeth? You know - the doctor's wife," asked Mrs. Grainger. "She glints, just a little, when she smiles. I think she has gold in her eye teeth."

Indeed, I had seen Mrs. Davenport's teeth. It was I who had placed the gold there. She had come to my surgery complaining of some sensitivity in her upper canines. When I inspected them, I found they were decaying along by the gum line and needed filling.

"Is it possible for you to fill them with gold?" asked Mrs. Davenport. "I don't want to dazzle people, but I have always liked just a little gold showing when a person smiles. Not much more than a hint. What do you think?"

And so Mrs. Davenport had some discreet gold fillings placed in her upper canines, high along the gum line. And when she smiled at Mrs. Grainger, there was just a hint of gold. And Mrs. Grainger noticed. And she wanted some too.

So Mrs. Grainger had some discreet gold fillings placed high in *her* canines, and when she smiled, there was the hint of a glint. I wonder what Mrs. Davenport thought! But Mrs. Bellamy-Rose noticed them when Mrs. Grainger smiled at *her* during a meeting of the local Women's Institute. So she came to me to enquire.....

It could be called a chain reaction, or domino effect. And it really became quite fashionable in our little town, for ladies to sparkle.

* * *

Maybe the hint of a glint could be seen as tasteful. Even sophisticated. But in some cultures, the flashing of gold from the oral region speaks of status and wealth. As related in the previous chapter, I was in the old Soviet Union in the winter of 1986/87, shivering a little from the chill in the air that accompanies thawing snow, and hoping that the lift (*elevator* to my American readers) would not be too long arriving. But there was a small crowd waiting. The lift arrived, and without even waiting for people to get out, those who had gathered started pushing in. Those at the back were actually pushing those in front of them. Manners! Some had their mouths open in what appeared to be snarls, and there under their Mongolian high cheeks, were golden mouths. The upper front teeth of several of the pushers, and those fighting to get out, were crowned with gold.

Neither the scrum around the open lift doors, nor the golden snarls, would be acceptable in England. So my wife and I stood back, politely but unnoticed, and waited for the next lift which, thankfully, we had to ourselves.

* * *

Gold has been used for restoring teeth for millennia. It was found in molar teeth in a burial shaft at Giza in Egypt, making it around 2,500 years old. Today, teeth take up around 80 tons of gold every year.

When I trained, broken down front teeth had their corners restored with gold, or we used a porcelain crown. Crowns for back teeth were always gold, as porcelain was not strong enough. Then a technique of bonding porcelain to white gold and other precious metal alloys was developed, and tooth coloured crowns started being constructed for molars and premolars. More recently, stronger ceramics are being used for restoring all surfaces of all teeth, providing both strength and aesthetics. But I still love to see gold restoring back teeth, and believe it has properties that make it the material of choice for crowning.

* * *

Goldentooth - who paid for it? Sometimes the patient, sometimes the NHS, and sometimes part each. Occasionally it would be an insurance company. But the gold crown always *belonged* to the patient.

"Mrs. Rennie. Would you like to keep the tooth I have just extracted?" I would ask, and then explain, "It has a gold crown, and therefore some value."

"Urrgggghhhhh! Horrible thing," was a fairly predictable reply. But sometimes the patient would like to keep it, and I would sterilise it with alcohol and wrap it in tissues. I understood that a genial jeweller might offer around £5 on a good day. Having said that, the gold content of the crown had cost me many times that when I paid the technician for making it.

But most people were glad to see the back of a tooth that had probably given them considerable pain before exiting in the beaks of my forceps. After the patient had left, I would clean it and sterilise it, and pop both tooth and attached crown into a jar, hidden behind the closed door of a cupboard. Many dentists did likewise, and then sold them, teeth and crowns, to a scrap metal dealer specialising in dental gold. Some would come to the surgery with a small spring balance with which to weigh the glinting mess of gold and teeth, and some were postal. A certain degree of trust was involved (How much did they weigh? What carat were they? What was the price of gold today? What other precious metals were in the alloys?), but I had an interesting way of estimating the true value myself.

When the jar was reasonably full, I would take it home and wait for a dry, warm day. Taking a hammer with me, I would sit on our stone patio with the jar beside me. *CRACK!* The hammer would smash the tooth against the stonework, and fractured enamel and root would shoot out, skidding across the patio and into the flower beds. Usually, the gold was retained under the hammer. Bent, crushed, but retained.

I would place the pieces of scrap gold in a polythene freezer bag, and weigh them on my kitchen scales. Assuming that on average there was 75% actual gold, and knowing its value from the finance pages of the Daily Telegraph, I could estimate the value. And when the little man with the spring balance arrived, I would be in a position to haggle for the rather grubby bank notes that concluded the deal.

Stella Manson, a very pleasant lady from our village, attended to have a molar with a gold crown extracted. 'No, she most definitely did *not* want to take the tooth home.' After giving her post-op instructions concerning pain or bleeding later that day, I bade her farewell, and opened my 'tooth jar'. It was almost full, so I took it out to my car ready for transporting it home later. It turned out to be a pleasant evening, so after finishing supper, I went to my tool box and took the hammer and jar of teeth to the patio.

CRASH! Tooth fragments whizzed through the air, and a tiny piece of gold was retrieved and dropped - tinkle, tinkle - into a fresh jar. *SMASH!* Enamel and root skidded across the patio. I retrieved the gold crown. Tinkle, tinkle. Periodically I paused, and on doing so after about 20 minutes, I froze. Stella Manson had walked in through the side-gate at the top of the lawn, and was walking towards me. Fortunately, her head was down and she appeared to be holding a scarf against the side of her face.

I frantically brushed tooth fragments and dust onto the flower beds, hid both jars amongst the shrubs, and started pulling out weeds. As she stepped onto the patio, I appeared to be startled. "You made me jump, Mrs. Manson. How are you after your visit this morning?" I enquired.

"I think it's just reassurance I want," she replied. "Paracetamol has taken care of some aching from the socket, but it is oozing a little. As I live so close, I thought I would wander down and ask you."

"No problem at all," I said, leading her away from the patio and into the house. "I'm just pulling out a few weeds. Now, I keep a small mouth mirror in my study, so do come through...."

* * *

Not all golden teeth reach their intended destination. We waited for delivery of gold crowns from one local laboratory, and eventually phoned the technicians to make sure they really would be delivered in time for the patient's appointment. Alas, the laboratory had been burgled, and was such a mess they could not even find the paperwork informing them which dentists were expecting delivery of which items. And in any case, my gold crowns were gone.

But another sad story, which was not without humour, involved some gold crowns I was going to fit, being rubbished. Rubbished? - let me explain.

There was, in the city where I practised, a fish and chip man called Tony Wyman. One of his customers was a dental technician called Paul Baker. He was very proficient at his work, and had actually trained other people to be dental technicians, albeit in Burma. Paul was keen to expand his business, but needed capital, and when his local fish and chip man expressed dissatisfaction with his lot in life, Paul had a brainwave. If Tony sold his fish and chip business and put the capital into expanding the laboratory, Paul would make him a partner and train him to make golden teeth. If he could train Burmese gentlemen, then he could train a British fish and chip man.

I and my associates would take impressions of teeth prepared for crowns, and a technician from Paul Baker's laboratory would call in and collect them. However, their routine in delivering the crowns was a little unusual, in that they would set out early in the morning, often before sunrise, and leave a box of crowns and dentures on a window sill at the rear of the practice. This left the whole day free for them to get on with laboratory work.

We suggested that the gold crowns and other items were not secure sitting on an external window sill, but Tony and Paul assured us that they left boxes of gold crowns on window sills all over the city and county. Beside, our rear window sills were within our back yard which was fenced off, with a gate leading on to a path serving other gates to other back yards.

Few people used this path and the gates leading to the back yards - but the dustmen did. Dustmen? - I think their work title has changed over the years. Garbage collectors. Bin men. Whatever they called themselves, regardless of what others called them, they came and emptied our bins early, every Tuesday morning.

It was a Tuesday morning early in summer, and the staff were arriving at my city practice. Head receptionist Daphne came up to my first floor suite, comprising surgery, waiting room, and office/consulting room. She looked somewhat concerned, and explained that I had a number of patients booked in for crowns and dentures to be fitted, but that they were not on the window sill when she had arrived. I suggested she phone the laboratory and speak to the technicians. But even while Daphne was speaking to the technicians, Bert Robinson, who had the fruit and veg shop on the corner, appeared at the hatchway. He was agitated.

"I think you might be short of teeth this morning," he puffed. "It's the dustmen. They were really stroppy, and one of them kept swearing and saying, 'Everything goes!' What alarmed me was that he was carrying a box with lots of your laboratory packets and tickets. I said I thought you would need them, but he just said, 'Everything goes' and threw them in his rubbish truck with that big mincer thing chewing everything up on the back."

Daphne looked up from the phone. "Paul says they *did* deliver them," she said, looking extremely worried.

And then a man from further down the road came in, and he was not looking happy. He swore.

"B****y dustmen," he raged. "I left an old pram out for them this morning. They took my bin, but ignored the pram. So I went after them and told them that they must be blind, or lazy, or stupid. They had left the pram. I told them what I thought. But then the big chap who seems to be their leader, he went ballistic. He started picking up all sorts of stuff from my yard, like gardening stuff and the bike from my shed, shouting, 'OK boys. Everything goes.' I got my gardening stuff and bike back, but they were just taking everything they could see."

Daphne picked up the telephone directory and looked up the number of the local government department responsible for dustmen. She was soon through to them, only to be told the dustcart would be on its way to the tip. This was before the days of mobile phones or computers. Daphne phoned the technicians, who said they would drive to the rubbish tip immediately.

Apparently the dustcart had tipped all its rubbish onto the tip, which resembled a small mountain of... well, rubbish, garbage, everything. The leader of the pack was stomping around muttering 'Everything goes' and the technicians were livid, searching among the filth for the gold crowns and plastic dentures that had each taken hours of work to make. The situation was not helped when one of the dustmen, with a rather gormless expression, cigarette hanging from his mouth and coffee mug in hand, pointed at Tony and said, "You're the fish and chip man from Bogford Road, you are. What are *you* doing here, fish and chip man?"

After more than an hour of searching, the technicians had found just one gold crown of the seven they had delivered. Also, there was a plastic denture. A patient had brought it to me as it had broken into two pieces. The laboratory had mended it. But now it had been through the dustcart's mincer - and was in thirty-five pieces.

It was not a good day. Our patients felt let down, the technicians had to repeat hours and hours of work, and the dustmen were not interested. But from that time on, I gave the technicians a key to the practice, and they would let themselves in, leave the crowns in the office, and lock up on the way out.

Those dustmen had rubbished my crowns!

* * *

Goldeneye was, in the Bond film, a weapon that could cause tremendous destruction. Goldentooth? I have gold restorations in my mouth which resist destruction, that have been there for decades, and which will probably be carried out with the rest of me, feet first, one day.

Gold has served the profession well, and when properly and professionally constructed, crowns and inlays are virtually indestructible. Of course, I am assuming that the patient cleans their teeth properly.

Goldenteeth - I must have supplied thousands of them!

Chapter 8

For Your Teeth Only

Secrecy and discretion are integral to being a government agent in MI5. *FOR YOUR EYES ONLY* would have been stamped across numerous documents and folders that were handed to 007. In the Bond film, *For Your Eyes Only (1981)*, the final scene concludes with Bond (Roger Moore) and Melina Havelock (Carole Bouquet) in a bedroom. She drops a towel, and as the camera fades out, says, "For your eyes only, darling." Just what did she mean!

* * *

'For your teeth only' varies in meaning according to where you place the emphasis. 'For *your* teeth only' would refer to an appliance that was specifically for just one individual, whereas 'For your *teeth* only' would indicate that something was not to be used for anything other than teeth.

"Could you take your top plate out for me please?" I asked Mr. Harris as he sat in my dental chair. I had made him a metal skeleton denture with just three teeth on it six months previously.

"No," replied the patient, and opened his mouth wide.

"I'm sorry," I explained. "I need your plate out in order to examine your teeth properly."

Silence. Then Mr. Harris told me that he could not take the plate out. He had never taken the plate out because it felt so much a part of him from the moment I had fitted it. Now it would *not* come out.

My heart sank. The denture was constructed 'for his teeth only', and fitted precisely. But teeth move, ever so slightly, and now it really was impossible to remove Mr. Harris' denture. Except by drilling - through the metal, taking around forty-five minutes, being so careful not to slip into the roof of the mouth. And the stench from under it almost made both of us vomit.

Partial and full dentures are made to fit the mouth precisely, and will not fit anybody else. Having said that, I had one couple attend the surgery who shared a set of teeth, and ate their meals consecutively, passing the teeth from one to the other. They had done this for so many years that they could not remember whether they were his, hers, or somebody else's. And they fitted neither of them.

We take impressions of the mouth in very elastic, yet stable, materials. They are usually alginates, made from seaweed, or synthetic rubbers. When the new dentures are fitted, people sometimes think they will continue for the rest of their lives. But if they are going to live for more than a few years, they will need replacing. The ridge (where the extracted teeth used to be) shrinks, and the denture, or plate, no longer fits properly. Not only so, but it does more harm than good, and accelerates further shrinkage.

"My teeth are loose," said a lady for whom I had constructed dentures just a year previously. They certainly no longer fitted, and I could not think why. Until she told me that she had lost four stone through successful dieting. In fact, nothing now fitted; jackets, blouses, dresses, skirts - and teeth!

The simple passing of time, ageing, also results in gum shrinkage, as do chronic medical conditions. The teeth were 'their teeth only' but are now no good for anyone.

* * *

Cliff Benton was a comedian. Not professionally, and never on stage (as far as I know), but the 'everyday life' sort of joker.

"You do cosmetic crowns, don't you?" said Cliff, with more than a twinkle in his eye. "I'm really interested in having a little job done on my eye teeth." I enquired what type of 'little job' he might have in mind.

"There's a party next month," he explained, with barely concealed excitement. "It's going to be a right little shindig, and I'm going to get them really shrieking. With your help, of course. Dracula! Dracula teeth, that is. I'm sure you can do it." He gave a wink and a grin.

"Dracula teeth?" I asked, not quite sure what Cliff had in mind.

"Yeah! Dracula teeth. On the eye teeth. You can grind them down a bit, and then fit really big ones, can't you? Dracula teeth!" Cliff was becoming passionate.

So we discussed Cliff's proposed treatment, namely to fit large 'fangs' to the upper canines, to give him the appearance of 'the vampire to end all vampires'. It would involve cutting down sound teeth, and then fitting crowns that would extend down rather like walrus' fangs. Like Dracula, in fact. I was not enthusiastic. Why?

It involved the destruction of sound tooth tissue. ("Like all other cosmetic crowns," said Cliff). They would not enhance his general appearance, in the way that most cosmetic crowns do, I countered. ("But beauty lies in the eye of the beholder," responded Cliff). "They could traumatise the lower gums by biting into them," I warned. ("Then be careful," said Cliff, with an apologetic smile). And what if he soon became tired of handling them in his everyday life as an electrician? Would he ask me to make some more conventional crowns until the next party, and then construct some more Dracula teeth'?

But I really felt this was a treatment too far. Supposing, after a few drinks, he bit someone. Just for fun, of course! Or maybe, in the subdued shadowy lighting, a young female saw this vampire descending on her, and had some sort of seizure. And who would be held responsible?

I could also imagine the headlines in some of our more seedy national rags, as I was hauled before the Disciplinary Committee of the General Dental Council. *FANG PRANGER'S*

DRACULA BITES GIRL TO DEATH! Or, *GNASHER BASHER'S MONSTER MAULS MAIDEN!* But most of all, I really did not think that Cliff had thought through the implications of such a treatment, once the 'right little shindig' was over.

So I declined the invitation to transform Cliff into a Transylvanian vampire. However, he had his own solution. His upper incisors, all four, were already replaced with a plate, and so, at the party, he simply removed it. "Scared the living daylights out of them," he told me with a grin from ear to ear, like a gappy Cheshire cat.

The Dracula crowns would indeed have been 'for his teeth only' - but at times there are other considerations.

* * *

And then there are those who want the exact opposite.

"In the course of following my chosen profession," said Charlie Montague, with a pronounced local accent, and wearing a clearly bespoke suit that made an expensive statement, "I have sustained the loss of my top front teef."

Charlie was not a patient of mine, but of Harry Posnik, who was delivering a lecture I was attending in Cambridge, on private dental practice. He told us of how Charlie had presented as a new patient, feeling it was time he 'got his front teef sorted out'. In fact, he had no front teeth. He had lost his upper incisors years earlier 'in the course of following his chosen profession'. His chosen profession? – debt collector, though I am sure he had a somewhat more sophisticated title for it. Well, rat-catchers are rodent operatives, dustmen are refuse collectors, bookies are turf accountants, and a used car salesman in South London recently described himself as 'a pre-owned vehicle re-allocation consultant'.

So Mr. Posnik discussed possible treatments with Charlie Montague, who went for the best available. Today, that would be an implant, but back in the late 1970s, a bridge was the most secure and the most permanent. It would fit precisely and be cemented securely in position. It would be for *his* teeth only.

Through conversation during the course of treatment, Charlie spoke of how he had 'started at the bottom', but had been more successful than any of his peers. Even if it did cost him his front teeth! As a result, he was now managing director of the country's largest debt collecting company.

He was more than pleased with his treatment, and asked Mr. Posnik whether he would consider taking on the entire board of directors of Charlie's company. They had all worked their way up through the ranks, and were all well-off gentlemen; cost would be no problem.

And so around a dozen men in expensive suits came along to Harry Posnik's surgery. Some were tall, and some were short. Some were fat and some were thin. Some were bald and some had a good head of hair. But they all had one thing in common – none of them had any front 'teef'!

* * *

"Gum shields, darling," shouted Ivor Payne across the table, with a mouthful of food and a raucous laugh. A lady present turned red with embarrassment, while her husband went white with rage. Ivor Payne was a local dentist, a rogue who gets more than a mention elsewhere in this book, and who once was the life of the party at a dental gathering for dinner at my home. Let me tell you about it.

I keep reading that we need to be *proactive*, which means, I believe, that we should react positively to the situations life throws at us. I think I do so. Married for around fourteen years, with a wife and four daughters, I found myself alone. I was well looked after by a Christian family, but after six months of unsuccessfully trying to restore the marriage and family, I drew a line under it. Was I proactive? I bought a small cottage, redecorated it, bought chickens and ducks, had a new kitchen fitted, learnt to cook, and started giving dinner parties. After six to twelve months, I decided I was proficient enough to invite a few dentists and their wives round for an evening. Pete Swift and his wife were *avant garde*, high flying whizz kids. Ivor Payne was ever Ivor Payne. Other dentists and wives were present at table, as Pete's wife Zena, shrilly announced,

"By the way everybody, I have just started a small business constructing gum shields. Every colour you can imagine, and just £12 each. You can sell them for £35. You just *have* to come to me."

Gum shields were worn by sportsmen to protect their teeth, and were increasingly in demand by pupils of certain local private schools where rugby, squash and hockey were in the curriculum.

"Well, I'm not," said Ivor Payne drily, and continued enjoying the *boeuf bourginon*.

"And why will you not be buying Zena's gum shields?" asked Pete, clearly feeling his wife had been insulted.

"Because they're crap," continued Ivor, without even looking up.

Ivor Payne was not a popular man within the profession, being widely known for his coarse, and even obscene, remarks to patients. His dentistry was best left without comment, and he was eventually erased from the dental register - struck off - for unprofessional conduct and incompetence. But Pete and Zena were also unpopular, though they were oblivious to it. Pretentious, and always one step ahead of the rest of the profession, they had indeed honoured the likes of the rest of us by joining us for the evening.

Silence. Suppressed smiles from most present. Ivor continued chewing, staring vacantly into his plate. But there was an explosion.

"*Crap!* CRAP?" Pete was livid, and Zena had put her fork down and was trembling. Ivor seemed oblivious to all this, and continued chewing, staring, ignoring. "Why *crap*?" Pete continued.

"Because they're £12, darling," said Ivor. "Anything under £15 *has* to be crap. Don't buy them, I say!"

I thought Pete and Zena might leave, but they simmered down, and normal, almost, conversation resumed. Until Zena took off on another ego trip. "Guess where Pete's going for specialist training next month?" said Zena, glowing again. "Cambridge, for... *OUCH!*" Ivor had visibly jerked, as his foot caught Zena on the ankle under the table.

"Gum shields, darling. Gum shields!" said Ivor, without lifting his eyes from his plate. "Gum shields. Cambridge. Crap."

Red faces. Gasps. Suppressed smiles. And it happened once more. There was little further ego-tripping from Pete and Zena, and Ivor was for just one evening, a popular man.

Gum shields! They could be bought over the counter in sports shops, taken home and immersed in hot water, prior to being inserted over the upper teeth. When set under cold water, they would fit precisely over the upper teeth and protect them. Usually. Well, sometimes.

Or I could take impressions, and send them to someone like Zena (or a more reputable dental laboratory), where a shield to protect the patient's teeth was constructed. It fitted them alone. It protected them alone. It was for *their* teeth only.

Likewise removable orthodontic appliances, known as *braces* which straightened crooked teeth. They did not always work, and sometimes got lost. Why? Because little Marcus wore it in his pocket, and not in his mouth. They were for *his* teeth only, and his *teeth* only - not his pocket. Which brings me to the second emphasis.

* * *

The second emphasis is - for your *teeth* only. Not your nose, or your armpit, or your toes, and certainly not your pocket, but your teeth.

You might think that the toothbrush would come into this category, but No.

"Please can you check my gums for disease," said a very distressed lady, with beads of perspiration sitting on her brow.

She had told reception it was an emergency, and here she was. I asked why she thought there might be disease.

"Silly me. Oh, silly, silly me," said Mrs. Sadd. She went on to explain. "You see, the best thing for cleaning the toilet, in my opinion, is a toothbrush. You can get right under the rim with it." And then, almost in tears, "But this morning, I brushed my teeth with the wrong toothbrush. Horrible. Urgghhhh. Please check them for disease."

Toothbrushes are really for your *teeth* only, even if they can clean places that other brushes only reach with difficulty. But what sort should you use? I can remember the hard scratchy ones that I won at seaside Bingo as a youngster. Ouch! But at dental school we were told that hard toothbrushes caused bleeding, traumatised the gums and made them shrink. Manufacturers had listened to the profession, and those labelled 'Hard' were now, in fact, 'medium'. Likewise, toothbrushes that were soft did not stimulate the formation of keratin in the gum. Keratin makes the gum strong, and protects it. Again the manufacturers listened to the profession and soon all packages labelled 'Soft', contained a toothbrush with medium bristles. So what could go wrong?

"My gums seem to be receding rather quickly," said Mr. Rix, aged around forty. They were, and I could hardly believe it when I saw that even the root tips were now showing where the gums had receded. I asked him what type of toothbrush he used.

"Toothbrush? I don't believe in toothbrushes," said the patient. "I always use a wire brush. Always have. Scrub as hard as I can. Gets them so *clean*." And he took a lot of persuading to revert to a normal toothbrush, though he had already taken years, even decades, off the life of his teeth.

So, what sort of toothbrush is *best* for your teeth? 99% of dentists would tell you an electric one, and I would agree with them.

And toothpaste? If your teeth are sensitive, there are toothpastes to deal with it. If you are prone to gum disease, there are toothpastes to deal with that. If you want your teeth to be whiter, there are toothpastes appropriate for you. If you suffer above average dental decay, there is a toothpaste that will help you. So what do Wendy and I use? As it's the brushing that is important, and not primarily the toothpaste, we always use an electric toothbrush. I then consider the various toothpastes available, and select the cheapest. After a month or two, I use the next cheapest, in order to change the taste. A few months later, I change back to the cheapest again.

John Oliver founded the coolest hair-dressing salon in town. He called it *JOHN OLIVER*. So cool - and expensive. One of the partners booked in with me. He was a really nice guy.

"I've brought you a sample," said Simon. "Soap - but so much more. Wash your hair with it, shave with it, and brush your teeth with it." I did not!

Finally, for your teeth only, there is fluoride. If you are young enough. It was observed that children living in an area where there was a small amount of fluoride in the drinking water had less dental decay than others. Many studies followed, and, as a result, a number of health authorities started adding a small controlled amount of fluoride to the water supply, if it was not naturally present anyway. The fluoride combined chemically with a calcium compound in the enamel, making it more resistant to acid attack. Acid is produced in the mouth by refined carbohydrates, especially sugars, breaking down. Plaque holds the sugar, and then the acid, against the enamel. Over a period of time, during which this happens repeatedly (or in the case of some people, continually), the enamel is dissolved away and becomes porous, allowing microbes through to reach the softer dentine, which decays.

If fluoride is in the water supply either naturally or artificially, and is ingested by the child during the years while the enamel is developing in the embryonic teeth, that enamel will be more acid resistant throughout. Alternatively, fluoride gel and similar have been painted onto teeth by dentists, which improves the acid resistance of the surface layer only.

When fluoride was first added artificially to the water supply in some regions, there was an outcry from a small vocal minority. "It's mass medication. Today they are adding fluoride, and tomorrow it will be contraceptives." Why did the opponents of fluoridation so often suggest that mass contraception would follow? I have no idea, but so many of the opponents of fluoride argued in that precise manner. Our area did not have fluoride, and so we added it to our children's food in drops. Just a little. For their *teeth* only. To protect them.

Chapter 9

The Dentist Who Loved Me!

In *The Spy Who Loved Me (1977)*, Bond finds that an enemy agent, of the female variety, falls in love with him. However, it was a most tempestuous affair, as one would expect within his chosen profession. Dentistry, in comparison, is quite a mild business, but not without having those making declarations of 'I Love My Dentist' or - 'My Dentist Loves Me.'

* * *

Advertising used to be prohibited within the dental profession. Today, that has changed, though it is generally called *marketing*. But some of us always did.

"I regret to bring to the attention of the committee," said Barnaby Snodgrass with more than a hint of a hiss, "that a member of our profession has placed *two* brass plates outside his dental practice. He is in breach of regulations. *Two* plates."

Tony Baker was new to our city, and had set up a practice from scratch. He wanted prospective patients to know he was there, and advertising in any form was not allowed. So he did what he could, and as his property was on a corner, placed a brass plate on two of the exterior walls of his practice. And as Barnaby Snodgrass announced to our committee of the British Dental Association, this put him in breach of regulations, which stipulated that a dental surgeon could make his presence known by placing *one* brass plate outside the premises from which he practiced. *One* - and it was to be no larger than certain modest dimensions. "The local committee needs to take action to see that one plate is removed. *He is in breach of regulations*," said the indignant Snodgrass, who practised half a mile from Tony Baker - and who was haemorrhaging patients fast in that direction.

So how did people find a dentist in those days? We were advised to place a brass plate with our name, qualifications, and the words *DENTAL SURGEON* by the front door of the practice. It was not to exceed certain dimensions, and was generally around 11 inches long by 7 inches high. Plastic was deemed unprofessional, and likewise steel. The other way we were allowed to make our presence known, was through the Yellow Pages telephone directory, where we could have *one* entry - and not in a box. Just listed, with other dentists in the area.

But most practices relied on 'word of mouth'. On moving to a new area, a person would ask their neighbours or work colleagues, "Can you recommend a dentist?" And curiously, although dentists are generally considered to be hate-figures within the community, almost every patient believes their own dentist to be wonderful. This, of course, is a big generalisation, but let the reader listen to the manner in which most people describe their dentist. "He's different." "So gentle." "So caring." "Such a lovely man." "She's absolutely wonderful."

Marketing! Not advertising, but marketing. Advertising is the way in which you make people aware of your services or merchandise, and try and sell it. Marketing is subtlety different, and by contrast, simply makes people aware of what one has to offer so that they can enquire further if they wish. But that is *their* decision.

"Mr. Lawrence, we *all* love you," said the dozen or so attractive young ladies, radiating wide smiles. Perfect smiles. They were my city practice staff, and I had arrived one morning to find them waiting for me in the staff room. I entered unsuspectingly, to find them lined up facing the door, beaming at me. You see, each one had a large sticker on their uniform reading *I LOVE MY DENTIST!*

It was my first attempt at marketing within the regulations governing our profession. I had ordered hundreds (or was it thousands?) of large, bright stickers. Each looked like a football fan's rosette. Half of them read *I LOVE MY DENTIST!* and the other half read, *MY DENTIST LOVES ME!* We placed two boxes by reception, and patients (usually, but not always, children) would take one and display it on their lapel. Sometimes I would produce one in the surgery and place it on a child's jacket or blouse. They would grin at me. It was a very passive form of marketing, and I hoped the patients would see that news of my presence in the locality would disseminate widely before the local dental committee asked me to withdraw them. But they never did.

I think the Lord blessed me with something of an entrepreneurial spirit in those days. Or maybe I inherited it from my maternal grandparents and their forebears. The family business has been standing in the centre of the market town of Bungay for generations. Was it my great great great grandfather who started the business? As a youngster, my visits to Nana and Grandpa at Bungay were magical adventures. My great grandparents had lived one hundred yards from 'the shop' in a house called *Cransford*. I can vaguely remember visiting great grandfather, Ernest Wightman. He seemed very gruff, and I was told not to be frightened of him. Then he passed away, and Nana and Grandpa moved into Cransford, and eldest son Neville moved into the flat over the shop with his family. Drapery, haberdashery and furniture were retailed, and staff in uniform traipsed around the seemingly endless labyrinth of corridors and staircases. Everywhere was panelled - and a trifle dusty. Grandpa was Mr. Ronald, and my two uncles were Mr. Neville and Mr. David. From Neville's spacious flat on the first floor, two further staircases ascended to the second floor, where my mother remembered two maids and a nanny residing. The good old days. I think it was a successful business, and my grandfather was also an undertaker (mainly for friends, he said), and a valuer of businesses. He was chairman of the magistrates, and seemed to have held every office for every golf, football, tennis, etc. club in the area. President of Rotary, Town Reeve, and always a Feoffee. (Town Reeve? Bungay is the only town in England to continue with the Anglo-Saxon office of Reeve, who is a senior official with local responsibility under the Crown. Feoffee? Someone to whom is entrusted land or similar; a term dating from feudal times. In practice, they acted rather like a mayor and town council.). And Grandpa was such a godly man, with an open Bible in his study, a local preacher, Sunday School superintendent, deacon, and so on. I would walk alongside him, listen with awe to his wisdom, run errands for the business, play on his typewriters, and be pandered to by his staff. He would have been proud to have seen my dental practice grow from one ailing surgery to five thriving surgeries plus preventive unit in so few years. I think my grandfather must have understood something about marketing, though I also believe God generally prospers the righteous.

Now twenty miles north of Bungay, I introduced children's competitions into the practice. 'Draw a picture of your dentist' was always fun. I had red hair, blue hair, green hair, was skinny, obese, and always with a big smile. We judged the competitions every three months, and the top three prizes were a digital watch, and two calculators, which were all very new at that time. Everybody got a prize - and everybody told their friends.

Newsletters were not something you found in dental practices in those days - unless you came to mine. A short breezy article on some interesting dental topic, a cartoon, an update on staff news, and always a crossword. Having won some national crossword competitions, I enthused over compiling puzzles that were diagonally symmetrical and contained dental, as well as cryptic, clues. How on earth did I come to misspell the word *abscess* as an answer to one clue? *Absess*! A local headmaster still managed to complete the puzzle whilst pointing out my poor spelling. He, like every winner, received a year's supply of toothbrushes.

And very occasionally, when we needed new patients badly, we would send the prettiest of our nurses, with the cute little hats they loved to wear, over the road to the shops. Several times a day. Using the zebra crossing. Screech, screech... young men would be blowing their car horns, and whistling. We received quite a harvest of new male patients after such a 'marketing' exercise.

It's all changed now. In fact, I had a logo for my county practice. It was two molars, where the roots were their legs. They held hands and showed a welcoming smile to the apprehensive. A patient who made such quality signs out of hardwood constructed one for me, around three feet by two feet. We fixed it to the exterior wall of the practice, and I made him false teeth as payment. Recently, I heard of a dental practice where a member of staff dresses up as a six-foot molar and accosts prospective patients in the street. Perhaps there was something to be said for prohibiting advertising within the profession. Where is the dignity? It now sounds more like Disneyland!

In *The Spy Who Loved Me (1977)*, James Bond, surrounded by beautiful women, scorched around Sardinia in a white Lotus Esprit that travelled on land, *and* under the sea. I, too, was surrounded by fabulous (mainly) women (mainly). My staff were often beautiful, and nearly always very decent people. I loved them - and also drove a white Lotus Esprit, which would *not* have performed well under water. It was purely coincidental, but some of our patients jokingly called me James Bond, and my nurse Moneypenny. And if they had known that my credit card number ended in 006, and that I was licensed to drill...

Finally, on the subject of marketing, as a Christian I believe I am beholden to market my faith. It's called witnessing, evangelism, not being ashamed of Jesus, sharing one's faith, etc.

A predecessor of mine at the practice in Dorset was reputed to have had a Bible text on the ceiling. It was 'Open thy mouth wide, says the Lord, and I will fill it,' Psalm 81:10b. He said that when he tipped the chair back, it gave him an opening!

In my city practice, I had a small library of Christian books for several years. One man came to faith through them. I also had a poster on the waiting room wall. It was psychedelic, with the words *HELP FIGHT TRUTH DECAY - READ THE BIBLE*. One lady was really confused by it, and felt that Bible reading would ensure sound teeth, but could not see why.

I produced a tract which was an illustrated account of how I changed from being an atheist to a born-again Christian. I gave away over two thousand copies, plus tracts involving crowns, bridges and fillings. I had a sticker on my dental light reading *PRAISE THE LORD!* Today, I would be allowed to have a six-foot molar accosting strangers in the street, but might well find myself suspended if I started sharing my faith in ways that *were* permitted in my earlier days.

I love God. I love people. I love life. And to underline the fact that I really did love my patients (and my staff), many of them chose to demonstrate this with a large sticker reading *MY DENTIST LOVES ME!*

Chapter 10

Accomplices

Natasha calmly stepped out of her car, and walked slowly towards the blue door. She looked neither to the right nor to the left. She opened the door and entered the red-brick single-storey building.

"She's gone in," said the plain-clothed police officer in the unmarked car parked in the shadows less than one hundred yards away. "She's on her own now."

Natasha, a member of 'the firm' for several years, was in fact bristling with microphones and other electronic devices. No-one could have guessed. I did not, as she passed me in the corridor.

* * *

Bond - the name was James Bond - was not a one man band, but part of a team. At times he was a loose cannon - but without 'M', and 'Q', and 'Moneypenny' and a host of other people supplying him with information, support, equipment, etc. he could not have functioned. Likewise in dental practice.

The NHS is a powerful 'brand' in the UK. It attracted, and partly paid for, a significant number of my patients. Although quite a few of them came to me 'outside the NHS' and under a private contract, there was still a huge team of people on whom I depended, and who were valued more than they probably realised.

My team? When I bought my first practice, where my predecessor had seen a maximum of eight patients a day, I engaged a lady receptionist to greet patients, make appointments and take the payments. There was also a nurse, who though extremely pregnant, helped me in the surgery. She brought the patients through from the waiting room, charted their cavities on the records, loaded the syringe with local anaesthetic, mixed the fillings, and a thousand other things.

I am a born-again Christian. I knelt on the floor of my study at dental school in October 1965, and surrendered my life to Christ. An unfulfilled atheist became a very fulfilled child of God. And I soon came to realise that this was more than a 'belief' - this was a total change of life, experience, values, culture - as my Heavenly Father looked after me. My first five years in practice had been far from lucrative, but I had been more than adequately provided for. I had married, moved into rented accommodation in the town where I worked, and later arranged a mortgage and bought a small property. Two daughters had arrived, and we moved to East Anglia. I bought a run-down practice that we believed the Lord was directing us to, and braced myself for further years of hard work and modest income.

Modest income? My wife and I earnestly prayed about our situation, and patients just piled in. The place heaved with aching humanity. A ten-year loan was repaid in ten months, literally, and a second, third, fourth and fifth surgery were added in the first nine years. Team? I needed a team. There were the dentists I took on to work in the new surgeries, receptionists (my original Daphne needed help, and became our *de facto* practice manager), nurses, hygienists, cleaners, dental technicians, accountants, and so on.

So I gathered a team, and most of them were thoroughly decent people. I think that Natasha was - but she was wired up with microphones. And plain-clothed policemen were tracking her with their high-tec equipment. Let me tell you about Natasha.

I had started a branch practice in a small, attractive market town around ten miles from my city practice. Yet again, the Lord blessed me way beyond my expectations, and patients had flooded in. I added a second surgery a year after starting, and took on another dentist. He needed a nurse, and we took on Karen who was great. After several years she married, and a little later left to start a family - and Natasha arrived.

"You've taken on Natasha?" said our receptionist. "Natasha? Well, everyone knows her, and she knows everybody. Her mother is known as Fag Ash Lil!"

So Natasha became one of the team, and was trained in the art of dental nursing by us. She was a rather diminutive girl, and somewhat subservient. But soon there was a mystery.

"Natasha won't be in today," said Fag Ash Lil over the telephone one morning. "She's had an *experience*, you see."

"An experience?" I said. "What sort of... *experience?*"

"Let's just say, an.... " and I waited.... "*experience,*" said Fag Ash Lil. "An *experience.*"

It was clearly quite an experience, as Natasha did not turn up for work for three days, and when I phoned up to enquire, I was told yet again that she had had... 'An experience, Mr. Lawrence. You understand... an *experience."*

So when Natasha returned to the practice, I asked how she was, and enquired exactly what had caused her to take three days off work.

"I had an experience, Mr. Lawrence," she explained. "You know - an *experience."*

But I did not know. Some months later, Natasha arrived at the practice and acted very strangely. I was informed by another member of staff that she was "alive with microphones," and 'someone' was expected to come in and say things that would be recorded, and that he might be 'put away'. I guessed that she had had another 'experience'. However, the 'someone' did not turn up, which was disappointing for the rest of us, and we heard little more about the business.

There was one other matter of note with Natasha.

"She's in the club," said Emily, another member of the nursing team. "In the club?" I said. "What sort of club has Natasha joined?"

"No. *In* the club. Preggers," said Emily, clearly excited by such scandalous news. "So she'll be off on maternity leave, won't she? And we will all have to cover for her. Not funny. Difficult." I suspected that she had had yet another *experience!*

I told Natasha that I had heard that she might like time off for maternity leave, and enquired when she would leave, and when she would come back. But Natasha was now empowered. Subservient Natasha had learnt that she had *rights* and that *the law* said that *she* would now make the decisions. Help!

"*I* (with a big emphasis on '*I*') will tell *you* (emphasis on *you*) when I'm going to leave, and when I'll come back. And I'll tell you when I'm ready." And she turned and left the room.

The law. Bureaucracy. Rights. Experiences. Maternity leave. I was not used to this, but got the general message that the tail was now wagging the dog, and legally so.

After a few months, Natasha left us on maternity leave, and I was informed that I now had to pay her for sitting at home watching television as she waited for the next *experience*. Then one day she came to see us all, pushing a pram, and telling us that she had decided to become a full-time mother. She wished us well, and said Goodbye.

* * *

I was never quite sure how we came to take Trish on. My wife at that time was helping with interviews, and always reached out to the underdog. Trish was an underdog.

She was just about OK on reception as a helper. But she was a one-speed girl - and the speed was slow plod. Other receptionists would greet patients with, "Good morning, Mrs. Smith. How are you today?" Not Trish. "Are yer oilroight?" was Trish's greeting - if she looked up and said anything at all. So there was training, and we eventually decided that she was more of a helper, who would remain quietly in the background.

"Trish is crying, Mr. Lawrence," one of the nursing staff informed me. I went through to the staff room, where Trish was puffy-eyed, rather like the rest of her anatomy most of the time, with tears streaming down her cheeks and joining the rivulets of nasal secretions on her upper lip.

"It's my Nan," groaned Trish. "She's dead." She snorted, sniffed and secreted.

I told her to go home and see how she could help the family. She returned a week later, after the funeral.

"Trish is crying, Mr. Lawrence," said a member of staff. In fact, I could hear her bellowing in the staff room, and braced myself for the rather disturbing sight before opening the door and going in.

"It's my Nan," spluttered Trish. "She's dead."

Poor girl, I thought, losing both her grandmothers within a couple of months. I told her to take a few days off and see if she could help the family. She returned a week later, after the funeral.

"Trish is crying, Mr. Lawrence," said another member of staff, and I went to the staff room where she was bent double with grief, and secreting from eyes and nose. Apparently her Nan was dead - so I told her to go home.

A few months later we had a recurrence of a Nan's death, and again a few weeks after that.

Time for a chat, I thought. I explained that I had had two grandmothers, though I appreciated that in this day of rather complex relationships, some people had three or even four grandmothers. But Trish had been bereaved of five grandmothers in the past eighteen months.

"There're not my grandmothers," Trish explained. "There're my Nans." I still did not understand, and enquired what a 'Nan' was. She explained. Trish lived with her mother, and had never been introduced to her father. Her mother led a busy social life involving the local pub, and Bingo. She would make new friends, who would call round for a cup of tea or something stronger. And each one was called 'Nan'. The bad news for me was that for every Nan that died, a further three would come in as replacements. And the bad news for Trish was that she was having no more time off to grieve for Nans.

"Trish is crying, Mr. Lawrence," said one of the dental nurses. I entered the staff room to find the usual mass of heaving flesh and snot.

"It's my step-Dad. He's dead," sobbed Trish. I commiserated and told her to go home and be with her mother. But later the thought occurred to me, 'She's never mentioned a step-Dad until now.'

In fact, it turned out that she did not have a 'step-Dad'. It was the postman. The postman? Well, sometimes he pushed the post through the letter box and continued on his rounds, and sometimes he came in for a cup of tea. And when he came in for a cup of tea, he usually stayed for about three days. So, what do you call a postman who stays with your mother three days at a time? Simple! - step-Dad.

I found it easy to be critical of staff like Trish. But in what surroundings was Trish brought up? What values were built into her during her childhood? With regard to relationships, what did she regard as 'normal'? I would love to have helped Trish - and Natasha. I tried to show understanding and concern. Only the love of Jesus can really make a difference, and bring fulfilment into people's lives, so my wife and I shared something of our own story with folk generally. Most listened, some wanted to know more, a few seemed to make some profession of faith, and there were those whose lives were permanently transformed. I am not sure that Natasha and Trish came into the latter category, which is sad. Jesus offers 'abundant life', and those receiving him find a fulfilment in living that they never knew before, giving strength and joy, even when one is bereaved of Nans and postmen.

* * *

Everybody loved Jane - which was not her real name, but as she was known to all as 'Calamity Jane', I will call her that here. She was well-spoken, and certainly not Norfolk. Full of enthusiasm for her work, for people, for life, she brought fun and laughter into the practice and unknowingly kept most others entertained.

She told me at her interview that she lived around twenty miles from the practice, and that she had not passed her driving test. How would she get in to work each day? She told me that she would manage easily, and her sophisticated little laugh was followed by a mischievous smile.

Jane drove herself to work on her first day, and we congratulated her on passing her test. She explained that she had not passed, but would soon be taking it again. Again? Meanwhile, she felt she was quite safe driving in by herself. She laughed - and everyone laughed with her. Her humour - or was it a fun attitude to life - was infectious.

And then she appeared with a dent in the car. I'm afraid I've had another accident, she explained. Another? She told us that her partner was at times rather concerned about her driving, so when the driver of the car in front came striding back to speak to the driver who had run into his boot, she smiled and passed him her mobile phone through the car window. "Could *you* explain what has happened to my partner please? He won't be cross, and I've dialled the number."

She failed her test - looked concerned, and then laughed. Nobody would need worry, because all would be well.

The next accident resulted in her being without a front number plate, but she did not think it was too important. Until a police car pulled up outside the surgery. Suddenly Jane was gone, and we looked out of the window to see her moving her car, and parking it front end on to the external surgery wall. Maybe there was an inch between the car and the wall, and nobody could see anything at the front of the car. The police had only come as patients, and Jane smiled at them and calmly showed each of them in turn into the surgery.

Both she and her partner were enthusiastically involved in the Territorial Army. We asked her what she did there, and she beamed and said that she and her partner were on guard duty outside the main entrance.

"You have guns?" someone asked. "Are they loaded?"

"No. We are not allowed guns, so we each hold a broom over our shoulder," she explained with a chuckle. "Jolly good fun."

It was a privilege to attend their wedding in the south of England. Military uniforms, sunshine, a lovely setting, and an altogether beautiful day. And - Jane's car sported a new front number plate, and she now possessed a full driving licence!

* * *

Frank was a star, and again, everybody loved Frank. He was young and keen, and was greatly appreciated. But we had some interesting times that we now look back to - and smile.

I can still remember the interview. Frank came in, and sat down in front of me. I looked down at his application form, and looked up to find - where was he? In fact, he was striding past me, and heading for our rather basic surgery computer situated on the worktop behind me.

"Nice little job this. No trouble. Just leave this to me."

"Actually," I interrupted, "I am the one that uses the computer in here at present, though that might change at some time in the future."

Frank walked back to his chair and sat down. A likeable lad. Willing. Enthusiastic - almost too much. I told him I would let him know the result. He got up from his chair, turned towards me and said, "Well, praise the Lord." Praise the Lord? I felt that Frank had done his homework and knew that I was a Christian. He wanted to work at the practice. But, praise the Lord?

I gave him the job, and he quickly became a proficient dental chairside assistant. It was an unusual occupation for a man, but reflected certain changes in the culture and values of our society in the UK in the 1990s. This proved to be something of an advantage to both Frank and me when a training company asked if they could use us in a commercial that would be shown regularly on television. The practice was alive with excitement as the film crew arrived, and around ninety minutes filming provided three two-second commercials. They were shown on

Anglia Television almost every evening for around a year, and for several months at the Odeon cinema in our local city. "I saw you at the cinema the other day," would be a greeting used by several patients. "You were wearing your spotty bow tie, weren't you?" Yes I was. Fame at last. But Frank was the star.

We also had one or two less flattering happenings in the surgery with Frank. It was very early in his career when he handed the funnel to a patient, not realising that it had become detached from the hose. "Rinse out into there please," said Frank. The patient rinsed round vigorously, detaching particles of decayed tooth, saliva, old filling, etc. and then shot them out of her mouth into the funnel... and through it, onto her skirt. There was a loud shriek of hilarious laughter from Frank, and suddenly... he was gone. Amanda, our most proficient dental nurse, had extended her arm and with a deft flick, saw Frank hurtling towards, and out of, the surgery door.

On another occasion we had a very nervous patient heavily sedated, and yet still quite conscious. As a result, they shook around in the chair, and gave an occasional shout. Later on, as the patient slowly returned to a state of *compos mentis*, Frank passed through the waiting room and stopped to say, "My, we had a right little party through there, didn't we!" He had hardly finished the sentence when another arm was extended, and... Frank was no longer in the waiting room.

Frank knew I was a Bible believing Christian, and this led to some interesting conversations. One in particular will always remain in my mind.

"Ah, Mr. Lawrence," said Frank, pausing from filing some patients' records. He continued in a knowing sort of way. "It all depends which came first, doesn't it. The chicken or the egg?" I have forgotten what provoked the remark, but the conversation that followed was memorable.

"Frank – I can help you with that one," I retorted. "The chicken came first."

"No Mr. Lawrence," said Frank, and continued with great earnestness. "The chicken came from an egg, which came from a chicken, which came from an egg, and so on. Your 'first chicken' came from an egg, which came from a chicken, and so on. You see?"

"Wrong Frank." And I continued to explain. "The first chicken came from God, because he created all things, including 'the fowl of the air'. So back at the beginning, there was a chicken. God created chickens – not eggs. And that answers your question about the chicken and the egg."

Frank stared at me, trying to take in what I had said, and then asked, "Well, how do you know that?"

"Because it's in the Bible," I explained.

"OK," said Frank with a little smile. "Actually, I am reading the Bible these days, but I haven't got that far yet."

Memorable! After some years Frank left the practice to continue his career within the profession elsewhere, and we lost touch. But a year or two ago, we bumped into each other in the town where he had worked for me twenty years or so earlier. A week or two later, prayers started arriving anonymously on my mobile phone. Good prayers. Biblical prayers. It was Frank! So after all this time, we are again spending time together, but within a different context – church. Frank comes to our Christian Businessmen's meetings, and fellowship meetings, and has started bringing others with him.

"Hey Barrie," he texted recently. "What a blessing that you chose me from that interview all those years ago, and now we continue as friends."

A blessing to Frank? A blessing to me, and a blessing to our fellowship. I thank the One who sovereignly directs all of history, and who blesses us so greatly in the process.

* * *

And there were others who were not part of the team, and yet were so generous with their time and expertise.

Linda had been a dental nurse, and a veterinary nurse, and knew everybody in town. She drove a Volvo Estate car, and wherever she parked it, left the tailgate up revealing several golden retrievers challenging anyone to try and steal it. On countless occasions, Linda stood in for us at short notice, and saved the day. Linda was also a great conversationalist and it was at times necessary to interrupt her in order to get treatment carried out. Everybody - dentists, support staff, and especially patients - loved Linda.

There was also Simon. He went to the same church as me, and became a volunteer helper in my Christian bookshop next door to the practice. And if we were short of a receptionist or nurse, he would ask, "Can I be of any help?" And he could, and he was, and I was always reminded of this fact when I saw his dental records, with Simon's own writing on the front cover - *FREIND OF BARRIE*. Dear Simon, now working in the hotel industry. My *freind*. A *freind* forever. We are still in touch, and though Simon is now working in a very smart hotel in Malvern in the west of England, my wife and I called in and caught up with him just a few months ago, at the time of writing. He has promised me very favourable rates if we would like to organise a weekend away for our church.

* * *

Samantha Peters was a great nurse. She was not only proficient, but cheerful, energetic, and willing to help out anywhere. She was Bill's nurse, at my city practice, and though she was often to be found playing cards with him, probably would have been happier at work in the surgery. Also, she was trim.

And then my nurse left, and after interviewing a few hopefuls, we took on Samantha Gross. She had moved to the city a week or two earlier, having only recently met the man she now lived with. She had been living and working in Essex, but on the first day of her recent break at Billy Butlin's Clacton Holiday Camp, she had set eyes on Roland - and immediately 'fell in love'.

"He looks just like Starsky," she explained. "I just had to fall in love with him." *Starsky and Hutch* was a weekly programme that had the nation glued to the screen at that time. Starsky and Hutch were two American cops. They were handsome fellas. "But Roland looks like a rodent," exclaimed my associate Bill, the first time the man arrived to collect his new live-in lover at the end of the day.

Apparently he was a postman, but not your normal plod-from-door-to-door postman. Roly had class. Roly sat in a van. And Roly was *indeed* not your normal plod-door-to-door postman. Roly was switched on. He and his mate could do the day's post-round in three hours, and then - cards! Cards? They knew a little lane where they would never be seen, and after 3 hours work, they indulged in 4 hours of playing card games. And Radio One. And the odd beer and sandwiches. And a little snooze.

"Where's Big Sam?" asked one of the girls on reception.

"Ask Little Sam," came the reply.

I felt I had to step in at this point. "Excuse me," I interrupted. "Big Sam? Little Sam? Might I enquire who these people are?" Silence.

I felt that one of the two Sams would not be flattered by the name by which she was identified, but these names were now established. I could remonstrate, but it would still slip out...

"Has anyone seen Big Sam? Little Sam wants to ask her about some X-rays."

I hoped that a certain person would not cotton on to her name at the practice, but...

"I know I'm 'Big Sam', and it doesn't bother me. The other Sam is small. So there!" she explained.

And then another nurse left. Several applicants were interviewed, and eventually, a new girl was selected. I had taken little part in the interviews, having decided that the other nurses and dentists would offer valuable insights into the prospective new member of our team, and could interview and make the decision.

"What's the new girl's name?" I enquired.

"Samantha," said Sam. In fact, it was Little Sam who spoke, as we felt that Big Sam was too recent a member of the team to be involved in making such a decision.

'Samantha?" I blurted out. "Sam. Another Sam? What will this one be? 'Short Sam'? 'Tall Sam'? 'Hairy Sam'? Or maybe plain 'Sam' would be sufficient when compared with 'Big' or 'Little'.

"Maybe we should ask her," replied Little Sam. "Then she won't be upset."

So we did. And her response? Vicky! We asked if that was her middle name? " No," she replied. "But I've always liked the name Vicky, and that is what you can call me. If that's alright?"

Of course it was. And in fact, all three Sams were good nurses. Big Sam eventually moved on to work for another dentist nearer to the flat where she lived with Roly. Little Sam was still at the practice when, some years later, I sold it. And Vicky? She has a beautiful daughter called Amy. I was doing a little strawberry-picking on a farm near our home, when the lady on the next row called out to me. It was Vicky. Or Sam. She was doing well, she said. It was good to catch up in that strawberry field. That sort of thing happens in rural Norfolk.

* * *

I was so very blessed in having a great support team. There was a time when I had seven surgeries, but no partners. There were dentists and dental hygienists working in those surgeries, but the staff looking after them were tremendous. There were exceptions, but they did not generally stay too long. One young lady who took sick leave very easily and very frequently, and whom I asked (well, told, actually) to leave, reminded me of this fact every time I saw her in town by pulling a face and sticking her tongue out at me.

Sometimes treatments over-ran and the dentist had to continue working 'out of hours' at the end of the day. The nurse always, always stayed. I tried to reciprocate when a nurse needed time off for a doctor's appointment, or to watch a child in a school play. I introduced a bonus system based on the amount of work the practice as a whole was undertaking, and took the staff out to a restaurant for an extended lunch break a few times a year.

"Come on, Mr. Lawrence," one of the girls would pipe up. "Tell us one of your jokes!" And there was much hilarity and 'bonding'. The staff were fantastic. I continue to be in touch with a significant number of them on Facebook, through Christmas cards, and by simply coming across them in the area, and strawberry fields, and passing the time of day with them.

Chapter 11

Fellow Agents

When there is a Cold War in progress, some 'victims' just have to be removed. Taken out, in fact. But Charles took the wrong one out!

* * *

I wonder how often James Bond, 007, licensed to kill, 'took out' the wrong one. He was a most proficient, professional agent and assassin - and fictional heroes do not 'take out the wrong one.' But Charles did.

Up and down the UK, and indeed throughout the world, in our dental surgeries, there is a war on. It is a war on dental decay, gum disease, and poor oral hygiene. There are goodies and baddies, and I was an agent on the side of the goodies. I was licensed to drill, but at times had to take an offender out. Sometimes a local anaesthetic - a shot - would be required, and the patient's lip would go numb. Cold. Some might say I was engaged in a Cold War.

I have related already how my Norwich practice grew and grew. More patients and more surgeries meant more dentists. Not to mention hygienists, nurses, receptionists, cleaners, et al. And yet more dentists. The practice expanded rapidly between 1974 and 1982, after which it continued as a five surgery practice without further expansion, though I started a branch practice in a small market town around ten miles away. The branch practice was so small to start with that I jokingly told people it was a '*twig* practice'. It quickly grew to three surgeries. The most surgeries I owned at one time was seven, but that meant that I needed several dentists to work in them.

* * *

So, how does one find dentists to come and work at a practice? "You *have* to recruit internationally," advised a colleague around the time we entered the twenty-first century. "I have a Chilean, a Hungarian, four South Africans, two Australians...." But it was several decades earlier when I was considering how to find associate dental surgeons for my rapidly expanding city practice.

I had come to faith in 1965 whilst training at the London Hospital. Come to faith? An encounter with the living God - my Creator, and indeed Father through the atoning death of Christ on the cross - had radically changed my life and my values, and given me an overwhelming sense of purpose. I really wanted an associate who shared those values, and after my wife and I had prayed about the situation, I addressed a letter to the Christian Union at my old hospital, enquiring whether any Christian dental students might soon be qualifying. There was no Internet available in those days - and no restrictive legislation. The letter was passed to Bill Roberts, who had recently come to Christ in a similar manner to myself, and he telephoned me. We met briefly, conferred, prayed - and I had my first associate.

My second associate arrived in similar manner, though from a different university. Later I advertised in the BDJ (British Dental Journal). 'Dentist seeks Christian associate' was published and resulted in a few Christian applicants. Some time after that, I was informed by the BDJ that I was 'discriminating' in seeking a 'Christian' associate. So I then reworded my advert to 'Christian dentist seeks associate.' As I was not stating that I wanted a Christian associate - just an associate - this was deemed permissible. A few years later however, the same advert was deemed inadmissible. Why? Because it too could be interpreted that I was discriminating! Some years earlier, when I was a young Christian, there were those who were teaching that the days were coming when a secular State would make it illegal for Christians to advertise for fellow Christians.... "Alarmist!" some of us protested. But quite quickly, yet insidiously, it had happened. I dread to think what the future holds for practising Christians in this country. In certain occupations a turban is legal, but wearing a cross is illegal; quoting scripture on sexual values can result in prosecution in the courts; I think that further elaboration on this topic might already land me in hot water with the State authorities. But having said that, Christians must not compromise on Biblical values.

* * *

It was after I had added my fifth surgery to the city practice that Charles arrived for interview. He was not from my old hospital in London, and indeed was from well north of the proverbial line drawn from the Wash to the Bristol Channel.

It was a difficult day at the practice, as a dentist had called in sick. I obviously managed to create time to interview Charles, whilst helping reception cope with cancelling the sick dentist's patients.

"Mrs. Oversby has been cancelled once already," said Daphne, my senior receptionist. "And she is so eager to have her teeth out and dentures fitted."

A brainwave! The dentist coming for interview was properly qualified and insured (wasn't he?) and perhaps could show me his proficiency by standing in and looking after Mrs. Oversby. So, when Charles arrived, I presented my proposition. Did he go pale momentarily? Was there a slight stammer as he agreed to stand in for our absentee?

I entrusted Charles to my senior dental nurse, who went through the treatment with him. "Extract these teeth - any questions? And fit these new dentures - any questions?" No, of course not. No problem.

Some time later, I received an internal telephone call asking me to come to the surgery where Charles was working. Upon entering the room, I noted Charles standing behind the patient, who looked a trifle pale. Pale? - but Charles was ashen. He asked for a word, and whispered that the treatment had not all gone according to plan. I observed a pile of extracted teeth in a dish beside the patient, and whispered back, "Well done." However, as I turned towards the surgery door, Charles whispered loudly, "Wait. There's more." I paused, and he explained that the extractions had been difficult. I looked again at the heap of extracted teeth, and again said "Well done." I should add that the patient was elderly, and almost completely deaf. Her hearing aids were lying on the worktop.

As I turned for the second time to the surgery door, Charles again muttered "Wait." He opened the door and walked into the hall, where he turned towards me and stammered, "There was a problem." At this point, not wanting to be overly tedious, suffice it to say that after beating about the bush for a few minutes, Charles informed me that he had taken out too many teeth. When the dentures were fitted, there was a gap where one tooth too many had been extracted.

Keeping calm is an attribute that not all attain to within our profession. Generally, by the grace of God, I did. "Let's have a look at those teeth," I said.

Back in the surgery, I surveyed the gap in the mouth, and the pile of extracted teeth. Experience is useful, and I thought I could identify the tooth that should never have been there. I picked it up with my tweezers, gave it a quick wash under the tap (OK - not the level of cross infection control that one would expect today), and tried 'screwing it down' into the socket of the lower left second premolar. It seemed to fit. I tried in the plastic denture, and it looked as though it had grown there.

"Leave the denture in place for two days. Then carefully remove it, clean the area gently, and replace the appliance." I advised.

There were two memorable sequels to this incident. Firstly, we received a letter from the patient. As mentioned earlier, she was deaf and had been unable to hear clearly what we were saying, but we had been taken longer and been more fastidious than any dentist before. She wanted to thank us.

Secondly, many years later, another of my associate dental surgeons came to me at the end of a day's work. "Do you remember that elderly lady that Charles saw when he came for interview? Well, I've seen her today. She has just one tooth left now, anchoring her denture," he said with a grin. "Guess which tooth!"

I did not need to. It was the tooth Charles had extracted, and I had replaced in the socket. The healing process had 'anchylosed' (anchored) the tooth to the bone with new healing bone tissue. It would be there forever.

Meanwhile, I felt that Charles was basically a decent chap, and that the wrong extraction was simply a 'blip'. I took him on, and he proved to be one of the most proficient and industrious associates I had at the practice. Today, Charles is my dentist.

* * *

In Shaftesbury, I had been an associate dentist at Reg Carnall's practice. An associate? This was an arrangement commonly adopted in dental practice where the principal dentist, or partners, owned (or rented or leased) the premises, the equipment, and the goodwill in their entirety. The associate was self-employed and paid an agreed percentage of his turnover to the principal dentist. It could be a little more complicated, but it meant that in Norfolk, I owned the premises of my city and county practices, together with all the equipment and goodwill. With seven surgeries, there were quite a few dentists and hygienists, perhaps working there for three or four years before moving on. Some stayed longer and some moved on fairly quickly, and the responsibility to find replacements could be more than a headache.

In my early days, as I have explained at the beginning of this chapter, I took on dentists who were practising Christians, and who had a clear testimony of being born again. Why? Because I felt it would be helpful if we had similar values, and would gel together better as a team. In fact, we quite often talked and prayed together, but our faith did not ensure that we *always* flowed in totally perfect harmony. Later on, I would include an unbeliever within the team. "The rest of us are practising Christians," I would explain. "We do not try to force our faith on other people, but you might find you get invitations to meetings from time to time."

In fact, I really enjoyed the company of some of our unbelieving associates, and at times struggled with my fellow-believers. And they with me!

Glen Marks was not a believer, and one or two of my Christian friends expressed a little surprise at me taking him on. Well, he had green hair, cropped short. Usually green, but occasionally orange. And he was quite left wing politically.

"I see you have the U-boat captain working at your practice," said a dentist I was in conversation with at a meeting of the local British Dental Association. I saw Glen standing across the other side of the bar, pint in hand. With his long black overcoat and tall slim figure, and his head tilted slightly back, he looked exactly like a German submarine commander scanning the surrounding ocean from his conning tower, as portrayed in popular television programmes at that time. That was around thirty years ago, and yet only this week one of my former associates asked, "Do you ever hear from the U-boat captain these days?" I wish I did, because my wife and I really enjoyed his company.

Glen usually had a deadpan expression, and a voice to match. He always addressed me as 'Boss'. He had qualified about three years earlier, and then worked at a practice elsewhere in the county. He would arrive a little before 9 a.m. each morning, go to the staff room for a coffee, and sink into a chair, raising his Guardian newspaper like a giant screen to protect him from the world.

"Boss," Glen droned out from behind the screen one morning. "I think I need to talk to you. I might be going for a holiday with Lester Piggott." (Lester Piggott was a champion jockey who had recently been sent to prison for tax evasion). I asked what he meant.

"I expect you pay tax, Boss," said the monotone. I replied that I paid plenty of tax, and said I thought that Glen must do so too. Silence!

"Glen! You pay tax. Don't you?" I enquired. I pulled down the Guardian a little, and Glen shook his head solemnly. "Why not?" I asked.

"I haven't got round to introducing myself to those people yet," droned the voice. "I think they will put me away with Lester Piggott."

I thought about this as I poured myself a coffee. I pulled the Guardian down and peered at him again. "Glen," I continued, "Have you ever heard of National Insurance?"

"No Boss. Will they be after me too?"

I introduced him to my accountant, who asked him, "Do you have a box full of receipts and suchlike that you've collected over the last three or four years?"

Glen lit up, and almost smiled as he said, "Yes, I do. How did you know?"

"Because people like you always do," said my accountant, almost unkindly. He invited Glen to bring his box round to his offices, and Glen said he would. My accountant told me later, "He won't." And he didn't.

Glen invited my wife and I round for dinner one evening. His flat, which was in that part of Norwich known as 'bedsit land', had a deep layer of dust everywhere. Even over the piles of coins on his mantelpiece. He was courting a girl who was a student at Norwich High School, which was posh and expensive - but she was not around that evening. We had an excellent stir fry, and thoroughly enjoyed his company. Maybe Lester Piggott would too.

Two further years had passed when Glen gave notice and left. The dentists and the staff loved Glen, and we were sorry to see him leave. So were his patients.

Around two years later, I had a telephone call from an accountant in another part of the U.K. "Did Glen Marks work for you?" she enquired. I said that he had. "Well, he has come to my office carrying a box packed with receipts, and talking about Lester Piggott, and I am wondering if you can help?"

Glen - not his real name, but he will recognise himself here - do get in touch sometime, as we would love to catch up with you.

* * *

Tom Evans was another unbeliever that I took on as an associate. He was Welsh, loved rugby, loved cars, loved teeth, so he told me. He placed a large photograph of a Porsche on his surgery wall. "Motivation," he explained.

But there were problems. He seemed to ignore obvious cavities in teeth. He extracted teeth, but left so much behind that my other associates 'extracted them again' later. I asked to have a chat with him, and enquired whether these things were true. He was a large muscular man - but he broke down and wept. He said he would like to return to Wales to consider his future. A week later he came back, telling me he had decided to change his ways and act more responsibly. But he did not, and two or three weeks later left the practice by mutual agreement.

It was a year after Tom had left. "Hey Barrie. Guess what?" said one of my young associates. "A patient who used to see Tom Evans came in today. Tom had claimed the fee for extracting a tooth, but there was so much left in the gum, that I've crowned it!"

* * *

Bill Roberts was one of my first associates. He came straight from dental school, and had recently become a Christian. We would get on fine, I thought - he was a Christian. He would work hard, I thought - he was a Christian. He would really care for the patients, I thought - he was a Christian.

He arrived at our home, as he was a bachelor and we thought it would be mutually beneficial for him to live with us for his first few months. We showed him his room, and he took his cases up. The door of his room closed. My wife and I sat downstairs, when - "Was that thunder?" I asked. She thought it unlikely, as the weather was quite settled. Rumble, rumble, rumble - it was coming from upstairs. In fact, it was coming from Bill's room. I strode briskly up the stairs, and knocked on his door. But he could not hear with all the noise he was creating. I tried the door, but something had been placed just inside the doorway, and prevented it opening. I went downstairs, and my wife and I waited. Eventually the noise stopped, and Bill came downstairs. "Any coffee going?" he asked cheerfully.

"What was all that noise?" I asked.

"Noise? Oh, that was me moving the bed. And the dressing table and the wardrobe," he said casually. "I like to have rooms *my* way, so I have changed it all round. Could you make me a coffee?"

In fact, Bill was a really nice, likeable, friendly chap. But...

But, he had not learnt to say 'Please' or 'Thank you', and patients expected it. We taught him, but he was a slow learner.

But, he did not like dentistry, and would take his nurse to the staff room to play cards. We would have to shout to him that several patients were waiting - and he seemed hard of hearing.

But, he could be impatient with people. After a complaint concerning a child he had slapped, I spent an evening with the aggrieved father, but finally ended up drinking schnapps with him, and gained a friend.

But, he was a scatterbrain. One day he cycled to the bank to pay in his takings, stopping off at several shops on the way. By the time he reached the bank, all the money had fallen out of the trouser pocket where he had placed it. He did not know how much money he had lost. He could not remember his route through the city, or which shops he had been to. So the police sent two cars out to search for his money, and found one five pound note and one cheque for three pounds and fifty pence. I think that some people in Norwich must have thought Christmas had come early as they followed this lucrative paper-chase through the streets of the city.

But, he eventually came to me and explained that he felt 'called' to work with children, a position with the school dental service had come up, and though his contract said he would give me six months notice, he would be leaving in one month, because 'he had prayed about it.'

Christian? The slapped child? Called to work with children? But to insist that he honoured his contract would have resulted in a disagreeable dentist losing the practice goodwill fast. I wished him well, and suspected that the school dental service would quickly promote him out of the surgery, and put him safely behind a desk.

However, Bill had been a good friend. Whilst living with us, my children had enjoyed his company. At Christmas, Daphne our receptionist, would play piano and Bill would play clarinet, and the staff and our families would sing carols heartily before feasting together in true Christmas style. There were times when I had challenges to face, and Bill would listen to me, and we would pray together.

I came to realise that Christians can often expect too much from each other. We are 'a work in progress' and each one of us is on a journey. Bill felt I had let him down in some ways. I did not tell him that I thought he had his shortcomings. After he left, I never heard from him again. I have tried to trace him, but to no avail. Bill (not your real name, but you will recognise yourself here), do get in touch if you read this.

* * *

Nick Read (was it pronounced *Reed* or *Red*, some asked) was a really great guy. Friendly. Caring. Honest. Hard-working. We did not get to know him as well as some, because he was married and never lived with us like most of the others. However, he too 'felt led by God' to ignore the six month notice clause in his contract. There was an associate position going in Nottingham, and he 'had prayed about it, and so had the small group at his church.' God was telling him not to honour his contract - and he went! I felt a little upset and disillusioned - but then thought about my own failings. We are all a mixture. We are each on a journey.

Why was there a six month notice clause in associates' contracts? Because we booked patients in six months ahead, and so there was always six months of patients expecting to see *that particular dentist*. When I gave notice at the practice in Dorset, I did so six months before I intended leaving. The practice owner could not get a replacement within the six months, and so I stayed a little longer, having spoken to the dentist I was buying the practice from in Norfolk. It never occurred to me to 'pray about it' and break my contract.

* * *

Another of my Christian associates had a name that, for many of us, would have been unpronounceable. He was Oriental, and hailed from Kuala Lumpur, so he changed it to an English name, and did not even try to get us to address him in his native language. He was an excellent, caring dentist, and a good friend to me. But there was a slight problem concerning his new English name. 'Raymond Loo'. It still had an Oriental ring to it, but that was not the issue. You see, I had the dentist's name written on their surgery door, so that patients knew they were going into the right room. Raymond's surname was *Loo*. So I told him that if someone with a desperate look on their face walked in, and then appeared totally bewildered...

After a year or so, Mr. Loo got married. His wife was a beautiful Oriental girl. She insisted on cooking for him every day, as one might expect. And suddenly no-one was complaining about any 'dental smell' in his surgery. But if you did not like to spend time in an atmosphere incredibly charged with garlic, then that was not the surgery in which to have your teeth checked.

* * *

I had taken Bill on as my first associate, but there was still too much work walking in through the front door. I had been working there for less than two years, but it seemed that a third surgery, and dentist, was needed. I wrote to the Christian Unions at a number of dental schools, asking if anyone approaching qualification was interested in working with me in Norwich. Almost by return, there was a reply from Scotland that Andy Reid would like to come and view the practice. Panic. There was no surgery; just a damp room with wall-paper peeling off the walls. What a diplomatic man Andy was. Looking round that dismal, damp, miserable room, he said, "It's the right size for a surgery." And so I pulled out all the stops, and a few months later, Andy qualified and arrived in Norwich, and I had had the room decorated and fully equipped as a surgery.

Andy lived with us for a few months, and the children loved him. There was a television puppet called Andy Pandy - and my children called him Pandy. He was a good friend, and still is. We play golf together occasionally, and reminisce on the forty or so years we have known each other.

* * *

It was in March 1984 that I started a branch practice in the small market town where a family had been so kind to me following the break-up of my marriage the previous year. It had seemed an impossibility to expand at that time, but born-again Christians often do whacky things, because they feel that God is with them. My accountant told me I had a 50% chance of bankruptcy - but I proceeded with the project. Would patients come? Would there be enough work? I would need to support my wife and four daughters who no longer lived with me - would I make ends meet?

God is so good! Do you know that? My small branch practice rapidly became so busy that I could not cope. I advertised for an associate dentist, and John Midgley replied, and drove down from Derby in his ageing Peugeot 604. He seemed, and proved, ideal, and was soon an integral part of the practice.

We became good friends, having a lot in common, and two things in particular. Firstly of course, we were brothers in the family of God, and shared similar values. Secondly, we both had a wicked sense of humour. Wicked? - well, you probably know what I mean, but let me give you some examples.

"Mr. Midgley has really been making a hole in that tin of biscuits Mrs. Clithero brought in for the staff room," said Amanda one day - and immediately I had an idea. I thought it was fun, but some would call it 'wicked'. I sent Karen to the nearby shops, and she returned with two packets of fruit pastilles. I undid all the wrappings and emptied them onto a plate. With my syringe fully loaded with lignocaine hydrochloride, our local anaesthetic solution, I gently injected the solution into each of the pastilles.

"Don't touch the pastilles on the plate in the staff room, and don't tell anyone they've been injected with local anaesthetic," was the word that went round the practice.

John arrived, to be told by his nurse Karen, "There are some fruit pastilles in the staff room, but they are for *everybody*, so don't take too many." Of course he wouldn't, he told her.

Strangely, although everybody (except John) knew the pastilles were loaded, they vanished remarkably quickly. Karen remarked on it to John, who said he had enjoyed the occasional pastille when passing through the staff room. "Do you know what Mr. Lawrence did to them?" she said, as if confiding in him. "He injected each one with anaesthetic in front of us. I can't think who has eaten so many."

"You're joking," said John. "You *are* joking, aren't you?"

"Ask Amanda," Karen replied. "She was there too."

John asked Amanda, paused, and then proceeded rapidly to the Christian bookshop next door, where Dave, the manager, regularly prayed for the sick and afflicted. There was considerable mirth amongst the staff, but a few millilitres of local anaesthetic in the stomach would not cause any real problems.

And, of course, John was probably a greater joker than anyone else around. He had a superb sense of humour, and wrote the script for a pantomime staged at our local church, which was hugely enjoyed by the several hundred who attended. But his most memorable joke was really quite sophisticated.

"I bet you haven't seen one of these before," said John. "It's in the back of my car. Come and have a look." Together with my wife, two nurses, our receptionist and assistant receptionist, I strolled out to the car park. John opened the back of his car to reveal a substantial wooden cage. It was probably around a metre and a half long, and a metre wide, made of heavy duty wood. There was a run enclosed by stout wire netting at one end, with what looked like a fully boxed in sleeping compartment at the other. Stamped on the outside of the wood in large letters, were the words *DANGER - MONGOOSE*.

"It's a joke, John," I said smiling. "Looks fabulous though. Who are you going to fool with that? I say, take it in the bookshop."

"No. It's real," said John. "I got it yesterday. Always wanted one. It's in the sleeping compartment. It's dangerous, but it's shy. Don't put your fingers near the wire." And he started gently tapping the wood over the sleeping compartment, and saying softly, "Come on. No-one's going to hurt you. Come on out." A half-eaten hen's egg was sitting in the straw covering the floor of the run.

A furry tail appeared at the entrance to the sleeping compartment, and moved a little. There was rapt attention from each of us. Our eyes were riveted on that little doorway from the run where the tail had appeared. "Whatever you do, don't put your fingers near the wire," said John. "They really are dangerous." Everybody took a step back from the cage, but every eye was still fixed on the tail. "And don't touch this door, which is where we put him in," said John, pointing to a door in the wood at the end of the cage. But as John pointed to the door, his finger inadvertently touched it. There was a SNAP! The door flew open and a mass of grey fur shot out, flying over the shoulders of the little group of us staring through the netting. I think each one of us screamed, and two or three of the ladies started running as fast as their feet would take them. John was doubled up laughing - and strode across the car park to retrieve the large mock furry tail that the spring inside the contraption had ejected over our shoulders when, having got us in the 'right position', he had hit the release mechanism to fire it out. My heart was beating fiercely, but we had to admit that it was one of the best practical jokes we had ever seen. John proceeded to visit the dentists who worked at my city practice, and with whom he was of course friendly, and gave them the same treatment. The wife of one of them raced away shrieking, vanished round the corner of the street and was gone. Her husband said it took him twenty minutes to find her and assure her it was safe to come back.

We all loved John, and when, after many years, he decided to leave us and return to his native Derbyshire, we were sad. And not least his patients, who appreciated him far more than he probably realised. Today John lives and works in the USA, but returns to Norfolk most years. We often meet up during these times, and a few months ago (at the time of writing) John came to a party we were giving at our home, and met up again with Frank, who had nursed for him years before. "Your face is familiar," said John, "but I can't put a name to it." Frank, who has a little less hair these days, grinned broadly.

But dentistry has changed. Half a century ago, when I first entered the profession, some of us stood in those historic and dignified rooms at the Royal College of Surgeons in Lincolns Inn Fields, and took the Hippocratic Oath. Most of the profession practised it anyway. The oath? - that we would always put the patients' needs and best interests first, and live and work that way. Today, I believe that has changed. In general (and I know there are exceptions), young dentists wish to be known as 'professional', but the ethos of many is different. In my opinion, the 'bottom line', meaning 'profit', has become the dominant factor in running many practices. What once was a profession has become to many, but not all, primarily a business, and the businessmen primarily look after themselves. Alas, the profession is no longer what it used to be when I was 'licensed to drill'.

* * *

For years there had been two categories of personnel in dental practices, namely clinical (dental surgeons and dental nurses) and non-clinical (mainly receptionists, book-keepers, and technicians)

Early in 1975, Bill Roberts announced unilaterally that he was going to stop working on Wednesdays. I knew he did not enthuse about 'work' and spent too much time in the staff room, except when a tax bill arrived. We all knew when this had happened, as he would arrive at the practice ashen-faced and asking that more patients be booked in with him. Overnight, he would seem to lose all interest in playing cards in the staff room with his nurse, and start to act like a proper dentist. But after a week or two...

Also, early in 1975, I received a letter from a lady called Jo Taylor. She was a dental hygienist (did I know what they were?), and enquired whether I might consider employing one (did I know what they did?). I arranged an interview, though I was ignorant concerning their place in the dental team. Team? - that was *me*, wasn't it! But she explained that they monitored gum health, scaled and polished teeth, gave oral hygiene instruction, motivated patients, etc. She was clearly professional, as well as being a very pleasant lady. I decided she could be a useful member of our team, and asked her to practise in Bill's surgery on Wednesdays. "And what if *I* want to work there?" enquired Bill. "Give me six month's notice, and you can," I replied. Maybe Bill would consider changes to his own working week more professionally in future - and at least consult me.

Jo proved to be a great asset to the practice, taking that side of the work off my hands, and being so proficient at what she did. When she moved on, I took on Jinny, a practising Christian married to a former dental hygienist, who was by then a curate. She worked for me for years. I had a decent microscope placed in the new dental health education unit I had added, and when our dental health educator showed patients the bacteria in their plaque, they would ask, "What can I do about *that*?" - and be shown through to the hygienist. The dental education unit made a loss financially (partly offset by fees paid for sessions with the dental hygienist) but was of great benefit to our local community and their teeth.

After a year or two in my new branch practice in the county, I advertised for a dental hygienist to work there. A number responded, but the leader of the pack was Derek. By a mile. I interviewed him, but felt that perhaps *he* should have interviewed *me*. After training and working with the Royal Air Force, Derek had been with the Foreign Office, looking after the dental health of British ambassadors and diplomats around the world. Then the space race had taken off, and Helen Sharman from Sheffield was going to be the first British woman in space, orbiting the Earth with the Juno Space Project team. Derek soon found himself in Moscow, and then with Juno. Now - he was being interviewed by me, and later said he had felt apprehensive. Well, so had I!

Derek was more proficient than many dentists I knew. Patients travelled significant distances to see him, and he also taught dentists on courses where they learnt about gum surgery. We were good friends, and my wife and I were sad that he had to retire early due to a progressive, degenerative muscle condition affecting his hands. We later visited him at his retirement home abroad, and engaged Ged as hygienist at the practice. Ged had been trained by Derek, and continues to be hygienist for Wendy and me now that we have retired.

It is well over forty years since I was an associate in that dental practice in Dorset. Since then, I have had a significant number of associates work for me. With just the occasional exception, they were professional, conscientious people. They were also decent chaps. And they were my friends. What a privilege to have alongside me so many wonderful people who, like me, were 'licensed to drill'.

Chapter 12

The Opposition

James Bond, 007, licensed to kill, had an arch enemy, Ernst Stavro Blofeld. Blofeld was No.1 in the organisation *SPECTRE*, which stood for Special Executive for Counter-Intelligence, Terrorism, Revenge and Extortion.

Dentists have their own enemy, which could also be known as *SPECTRE* - Sugar Products, Exploitation of Chocolate and Toffees causing Rotting and Extractions. It was only during my lifetime that the connection between sugar and dental decay became clear. I have already stated that when I was very young, sugar was no more linked to dental decay than smoking tobacco was to lung cancer. But that has changed, and in general, eating sweets between meals and the associated dental decay has been dramatically reduced, especially amongst the middle classes. The same can be said for smoking and lung cancer. But for all my working life, sugar has been the dentist's No.1 enemy. It has provided lots of work for us (as *SPECTRE* did for Bond and MI5), but as a profession, we wanted to eradicate decay for the benefit of our patients (and likewise Bond and MI5 with regard to *SPECTRE*, for the benefit of the people of the free world).

However, there was a sense in which other *dentists*, and particularly those practising in close proximity, might be lightly referred to as 'the opposition'. In the small county town where I worked, there was another dentist in practise around four hundred yards away. We occasionally referred to him, tongue in cheek, as 'the opposition'. Also within the same town were two ironmonger's shops. I asked the proprietor of one how he felt about having another, more recent ironmonger, so close. "He is my greatest asset," he replied. "They are so incompetent and muddled, that I hope they never close down. Never."

We had a similar situation when I practised elsewhere in England. There was another dentist in the town, with a rather posh name, who was blind in one eye and rarely sober after noon. He practised from his dining room, and it was said that if he opened the top drawer of his sideboard, there were in order, knives, forks, spoons, mirrors, probes and tweezers, and forceps in the next drawer down. Not the level of cleanliness and sterilisation that is expected today! Once a year, this elderly dentist would apply to stay registered in our area, and the dentist I worked with was on the committee that considered such applications.

"Don't refuse him," my colleague would say, and add words to the effect that this gentleman was *our* greatest asset.

But over the years there have been a number of occasions when another member of the profession has been responsible for extra patients coming to see me, and so could perhaps be viewed as an *asset*. In my early days in Norwich, I often heard about the dentist referred to by patients as 'the hippie' or 'the beatnik' or 'the bloke with the long hair.' Apparently, as this gentleman leant forward to examine the patient's teeth, hair would fall, clump by clump, onto the patient's face, and periodically, the dentist would jerk his head to send it back over his shoulders. In those days, we still had the slow drill attached to a pulley system, where cords ran over a jointed arm. The motor was remote from the drill, and the moving cord transmitted movement to it. More than one patient arrived with the story of the dentist's hair landing in the cord, and of his head being yanked up to the next pulley. Ouch! But patients did not like his hair across their face. "So I've come to see you instead, Mr. Lawrence."

And then we had a succession of patients, literally scores,

coming from a practice several miles away, and each repeating one of two stories that we heard over and over again. An elderly, much-loved dentist had retired, and sold his practice to a younger man. The stories? They went like this.

"So he called me into his surgery and sat me in the chair, and then he said, 'How's that film contract coming along?' 'Film contract?' I said. 'I haven't got a film contract. You've got the wrong person.' 'What?' he said. 'Teeth like that and they haven't signed you up for Dracula yet? But for £500, I can give you a *human* smile.' So I've come to see you instead, Mr. Lawrence."

The other story we heard so many times was similar in essence. "I went into his surgery, and when I sat down he said to me, 'So how is the divorce coming along?' 'Divorce?' I said. 'I'm not getting divorced. You've got the wrong person.' He then said, 'What? Teeth like that and your husband's not divorcing you? But for £500, I can give you teeth that a man would stay married to.' So I've come to you instead, Mr. Lawrence." That was a long time ago, and £500 was worth several times what it is today.

One does not want to get a colleague into trouble, but I felt these people were being insulted, and could have been coerced into having unnecessary treatment. However, when I asked if they had considered complaining, they usually said that it would all get too complicated and unpleasant.

After some months, no more patients arrived from that practice with either of those tales. But around six months to a year later, more started arriving with a different story. They were all ladies, none of them skinny, and they all had the same complaint. "I sat in his chair, and he tipped it right back. Then he put his little mirror and other instruments on my... er... um.. chest. Then he leant over me leering, and said, 'I like big girls. Nothing falls off.' So I've come to you instead, Mr. Lawrence."

Another very obese lady added, "And I didn't like the way 'e pinched my bum all the way along that long corridor of 'is."
I found some of these stories almost incredible, and one or two

colleagues I mentioned them to questioned whether I, or the patient, was telling the truth. And then rumours started going around, suggesting that the gentleman was having to appear before the Disciplinary Committee of the General Dental Council.

But still the patients, and the stories, kept coming. "My dentist has just bitten me," said a somewhat enraged lady. "What?" I exclaimed in near disbelief. "He stared at me, and mumbled something about 'biting', and then he sort of pounced on me and bit me. Look!" she said.

Mrs. Fields turned her head to show me a red bite mark on the side of her neck. I was speechless, but when I found words again, asked what she intended to do. "I'm going to a solicitor, but in the meantime, can you please have a look at my teeth for me, Mr. Lawrence?"

I rarely came across the gentleman in question, as he did not attend any of the meetings of the British Dental Association, of which I was secretary for the Norfolk and Norwich Section, and neither did he appear to go on courses. However, a matter of days after the bitten lady incident, I encountered him in a supermarket.

"Just saved you from the law, old boy," he stated loudly, for all to hear. "One of your crowns dropped out, but I stuck it back in and persuaded the lady not to sue." He grinned, as most people within earshot stared at him, and then at me. I walked over to him and, keeping my voice down, said, "Trying to save *you* from the law, old boy."

"What? Come on, *my* crowns don't fall out, y' know." He grinned broadly again.

"I'm sure they don't," I replied, "but a lady has complained that you bit her. On the neck. Left a nasty mark. She has shown it to me."

The grin vanished. And then Ivor Payne (not his real name, of course) adopted a knowing expression. "Blonde? Petite? About 5 foot 4?" I nodded.

"Now look here," Mr. Payne continued. "I don't bite my

patients. Never have. *But* - if a lady comes in sporting a recent love bite on her neck, I'll sit her in the chair and say, 'Nice bite dear, but I think I can do even better.' I lunge forward and pretend. Just pretend, old boy. They love it. Shriek with laughter. Well, usually. But not the blonde lady. She just ran. Good riddance."

"Ivor," I said. "Suppose the lady does not know that she's 'sporting a love bite'. Suppose she's nervous and finds it difficult to concentrate on what you're saying, but hears the word 'bite'. You lunge forward and pretend, and when she looks in a mirror, she sees the bite mark for the first time."

"They love it," was the only response I received from Mr. Payne. And surprisingly, I heard nothing more about the incident with the blonde lady. However, Ivor's days were numbered. He seemed unable to empathise with his patients, and assumed that his outrageous sense of humour would be shared by everybody else, even though they were the victims. Furthermore, although receiving warnings and conditions (largely concerning his patients needing *always* to be chaperoned when in the surgery with him in future), he took no heed to the warnings, and ignored the conditions. Eventually he was struck off, but ultimately not for being offensive, but primarily for undertaking treatment at which he proved incompetent. He had hardly been practising on my doorstep, but we apparently shared a bus route - and he proved to be one of my greatest assets, furnishing me with hundreds of patients.

* * *

Another local dentist was an enigma to us. Andrew Holland was well spoken of by many people in the small town where my county practice was situated. And then, several of his patients jumped ship, and asked if I could take them on. Of course. But their gums were not in good shape, and I suggested they see my dental hygienist. "What's a dental hygienist?" they asked. I explained that he would scale their teeth. "What's scaling?" they asked. So Andy Holland did not scale his patients teeth. So they all had advanced gingivitis, and needed treatment. "What's gingivitis?" they asked.

Apparently Mr. Holland had 'gone private', and not all his patients could afford to continue seeing him. I have never understood why he did not scale his patients' teeth, but it seemed that the National Health Service were a little suspicious, and their breathing down his neck proved too much for him. He left the NHS and 'went private'.

So few patients continued with him that he then went back into National Health Service dentistry. However, after a year or so, lots more patients from his practice asked if I could see them. No trouble - but what had happened now? My guess was that the NHS investigators were getting too close for comfort again, because he moved abroad rather quickly. And another unusual aspect of Mr. Holland's practice then became apparent.

"I'll take X-rays of your teeth to make sure that all is as good as it looks," I told my new patient, Amanda. "Why?" she asked. I explained that this was the only way that I could see what was happening inside the teeth. "But Mr. Holland never took X-rays," said Amanda. "Never." Groan. The X-rays revealed that the lady had 16 cavities, and she burst into tears. I showed her the cavities on the X-rays. I accompanied her back to the waiting-room, where her partner saw the tears in her eyes, jumped up and said, "What's he done?"

"No," she said. "He's a lovely man. It's Mr. Holland. He did not check my teeth properly, and I need 16 fillings. I've seen them on my X-rays."

Her partner gave her a kiss, and came through to have his teeth checked. He too had seen Mr. Holland. Andrew only needed 12 fillings, after having his first ever X-rays. And they both had gingivitis. Andrew and Amanda lived in my village, and we became quite good friends, thanks to Mr. Holland.

Around twenty miles away, a husband and wife who were both dentists were in partnership. Their surname was Screech. Screech and Screech! I wonder if they had problems attracting patients. And then there was a chap I trained with at the

London Hospital, who had an immediate disadvantage. Andy Butcher! But you could not find a gentler or kinder man than the dentist called – butcher!

So there were a few cases where the 'opposition' proved to be a great asset to my practice. But they were few and far between, and the vast majority of dentists that I met during my thirty-five years or so in practice (and I met a lot, not least through the British Dental Association, our professional body) were conscientious, kind people, who put the needs and wellbeing of their patients above their own comfort or advantage. Most of us always saw people in pain the day they contacted us, and out of hours we turned out for people in trouble, and without charge or being paid by the National Health Service in my very early days. Maybe a few chaps, and they nearly always were *chaps*, had a different ethos from the majority, but those were the days when professional gentlemen were both professional and gentlemen.

Chapter 13

On Her Majesty's
National Health Service

On Her Majesty's Secret Service (1969) was the title of one of the James Bond films, based on the original Ian Fleming novel. I read it three times - like all the other James Bond novels. And I saw the film *more* than three times - the same as all the other original Bond films. But that was when I was younger, of course.

Bond was employed by Her Majesty, and worked, in fact, for the government. So did I - in part. Like Bond, I enjoyed working for Her Majesty in those younger days. But also, like Bond I suspect, I found that I really did not have the energy to keep up the pace as the years passed. And also, there were patients who saw it differently from me.

"I am *not* paying twice for my dental treatment," said Mr. Gardiner looking indignant. "I've paid for it once; I'm not paying for it twice."

Mr. Gardiner was elderly, tweedy, reasonably well-spoken, and felt cheated. He was typical of many of his generation.

* * *

Free dental treatment! That was what the National Health Service (NHS) introduced in 1948, and the population was told that all medical and dental care would be free for everybody. It would be paid for from taxation, and this was raised by expanding the National Insurance system that had been inaugurated in 1911.

National Insurance contributions were a form of taxation, paid by employers and employees, raised to help insure against sickness and unemployment through certain State benefits. In 1948, this system was expanded, and the people of the U.K. were told that they would no longer have to pay anything for medical treatment, dental treatment, or prescriptions. This was revolutionary, and suddenly, everybody wanted dental treatment. Well, you know what I mean! It was not a case of, "Please will you drill my teeth for free?" but more an awareness that charging for treatment no longer applied. Dentists were busier than ever before.

However, in 1951 after just three years, the government decided that the National Health Service could no longer sustain the flow of payments for dental treatment and prescriptions. For dental treatment, a charge of one pound was introduced, and for prescriptions, one shilling (5p in today's money).

Having qualified in December 1968, I started working the following month at a dental practice in Shaftesbury, Dorset. As a young dentist, all my work was carried out under the National Health Service, as those patients wanting to pay privately in order to receive (they hoped) superior treatment, would choose to be seen by a more experienced (superior, they hoped) dentist - and not by a young lad fresh out of dental school.

In those days, the dental examination was free. Most adult patients required some scaling and polishing, for which there was a small charge. Occasionally we took X-rays, which we called *radiographs*, for which there was also a small charge. But as soon as fillings were required, the ceiling charge of one pound (£1) was reached. It was worth a lot more than the same sum today, but patients generally paid without complaint.

Except Mr. Gardiner, and a few others like him. The government in 1948 had sold the population higher National

Insurance contributions by telling them, "Look at what you are getting for them. *Free* medical treatment from your doctors and hospitals. *Free* dental treatment. *Free* prescriptions." And when the government reneged on that, certain people felt aggrieved. And they usually made their feelings known to the dentist, because he was the person holding out his hand and asking for one pound.

Today, in 2016, I understand that patients can pay in excess of two hundred pounds under the NHS. One result of this is that many people decline treatment, or attend a lot less regularly. Which is rather like the situation prior to 1948.

By the time I retired in 2007, the NHS system had become extremely bureaucratic, with more and more forms, certificates, requirements, etc. One result of this was that an increasing number of dentists were ceasing to work under that system, and seeing patients solely under private contract. That too, is rather like the situation prior to 1948.

* * *

"Could I ask you for your date of birth please?" I asked Brenda Mayhew, one of the first patients attending my country town practice.

"It's the 3rd of February, 1944. I'm 40," was the reply.

"Oh no she ain't," reverberated through the thin partition wall separating the surgery from the waiting area. "She's getting on for 60, and don't you let her tell ya otherwise." This was followed by hilarious laughter!

I may not have been working for Her Majesty's Secret Service, but I was supposed to keep some things secret. Doctors and dentists, and most other professionals, are required to. Many things that I learnt about patients in my surgery decades ago remain confidential today. In my books, and when I am speaking, names, dates, places and other details are often changed in order to preserve confidentiality, as well as anonymity.

I had just set up my branch practice out in the county. The

city practice had grown to five surgeries, and was accommodated in two Victorian terrace houses that had been made into one internally. It was brick, and it was solid. My county practice was different.

Jack Ladd was no fool. So he told me when selling me the property. Jack Ladd knew the way the authorities worked, and he was shrewd when dealing with them. He told me that too when I bought the property.

He had acquired a plot of land not far from the town centre, and next door to the blacksmith's place, a few decades earlier. He applied to build a bungalow there, and permission was granted. So he built it. A year or two later, he applied for permission to build a garage next to the property. Quite a large garage, and around twenty feet distant from the existing building. Jack winked as he told me. Shrewd! Permission was granted, and the garage was constructed. But no planning permission was needed for a carport, and very soon after completion of the garage, a further roof structure straddled the space between the garage and the bungalow. And then walls appeared at the front and back of the 'carport'. Before long, Jack had a significant income flowing in from this conglomeration of buildings. The large garage had a shop window in the front wall facing the road, and was rented out to an antique dealer. The bungalow had become the premises of an estate agent, whilst the carport with walls had also become a commercial enterprise, housing a launderette where several washing machines churned away, keeping the town clean and generating revenue. Jack winked.

By 1984, the estate agents had moved out, and the launderette had closed. A dentist was working half a day a week in the premises, and they were closing down too. And then I was brought in. The dentist who was closing down telephoned me. She had heard that my city practice had expanded rapidly. I must have a gift for it. How about doing the same in the county? She did not want to sell, but just wanted someone to take this small 'three hours a week' concern off her hands.

I prayed about it. Well, Christians do. And I felt a peace in my heart about proceeding. But Jack did not want to rent me the carport-cum-launderette, now dental practice. "I'm selling the lot, and it's all three properties. Job lot - or forget it." Jack winked.

I prayed some more, seriously, and really felt this was God's way for me. I know that I can get things wrong, but I also know that I have to go with what I feel to be right.

I consulted my accountant, who told me I had a fifty per cent chance of bankruptcy if I proceeded. But I really felt to go for it. Banks and insurers were consulted, as I had no money, largely because I was going through a divorce, and in March 1984, Woodview Dental Practice opened. It was in the launderette, and this rectangular room was divided into two by a partition. The surgery was one side, and reception and the waiting area the other. It looked adequate. Yes, I could hear what people were saying through the thin board wall, but only just. There was no problem, was there? Until Mrs. Mayhew gave her date of birth. But she had an exceptionally loud voice, and so did her husband who had shouted his response through the partition wall. It was funny, but I realised that I needed to change the premises.

The NHS understandably required total patient confidentiality, as did the General Dental Council, the organisation that regulates dentists in the UK. The screen was too thin and I was in breach of regulations. How fortunate that only Mr. and Mrs. Mayhew were on the premises at the time, and that they were very friendly people, and members of a very friendly community. I loved the people of that town.

More and more patients piled in, and that August, I felt I heard the voice of God telling me to open a Christian bookshop in the town. OK, I will say it again - I know I can be wrong, but I had to go with it. My accountant became alarmed at this point, and suggested a name for the Christian bookshop – SUICIDE! So the dental practice moved into the brick-walled building, the antique dealer stayed in the 'garage', and I opened a Christian bookshop in the middle premises. And everything in the dental practice became more discreet. But what might have been vocal and amusing/embarrassing in the past, was now on paper as we increasingly used questionnaires when gathering information from patients.

'Sex?', was one of the questions on our pro forma patient questionnaire. The expected answer was either 'Male' or 'Female'. One simply had to tick a box. It was either/or. But not for Kevin Jones - he was 'Tuesday and Friday', and Stuart Brown was 'Wednesday and Saturday." And I am not going to tell you what Bridget Summers wrote!

* * *

Of course, there has to be some policing of a system like NHS dentistry, and there were *dental officers* who would come and inspect our patients. They were dentally qualified, and had been in practice themselves before taking up appointments as dental officers working directly for the NHS. There were two situations where we could expect a visit from one of these gentlemen. If we wished to carry out treatment above a certain financial limit, such as, say, ten crowns, they might be sent to inspect the teeth to see if it was really necessary. The second scenario where they might be expected was when we had carried out such a treatment. They would inspect the finished work to make sure it was up to standard. And sometimes, a patient would be chosen completely at random, and be inspected to see if the dentist was carrying out all necessary work, charging the correct amount, maintaining a good clinical standard, and so on.

Generally there would be two or three dental officers covering a region. A new one started coming to inspect patients at my county practice, and he became well-known amongst the profession in our area. There were no pleasantries, and he said very little to dentist or patient. He wore rimless spectacles, and was apparently known quite widely as *Gestapo*. And then he stopped coming, and a much friendlier gentleman arrived, telling us, "*Gestapo* has retired."

Another memorable incident was when the patient to be inspected arrived quite early during our lunch hour, and the receptionist showed him into the waiting room. The dental officer also arrived early and he too was shown into the waiting room. The two of them sat there in silence until the patient looked up and asked, "Have you got to see this bloke too?"

"No," replied the dental office. "I *am* the bloke!" He grinned widely as he told me about it later.

* * *

A number of my NHS patients seemed to have a slightly different vocabulary from my private patients. One of the words many of them used was '*abser*'.

"I've got an abser on this tooth, and it hurts like hell," was heard around once a week when I first opened the city practice and treated people from that locality. The nurse would catch my eye and give a little grin as she turned away. The correct word was *abscess*.

Periodically, I would take my associate dentists out to a decent restaurant for an evening, and we would simply have fun together over, say, Italian cuisine. Suddenly, one would say "Ouch", and appear to be in some pain.

"It's an *abser*," Chris would say loudly, and everyone would cackle with laughter. "I had an abser the other day," Glen would add, and then one of them would ask, "Who has had a patient with an abser this week?" Around half of us had, and one chap had usually had two.

Patients who suffered from an abser usually asked for '*penicillium*'. A casual listener at the practice might think that this was a Norfolk brand name of penicillin, but it was just the word used for the generic antibiotic amongst some of the communities in our locality. And of course, these same people often had *bronical* (never *bronchial*) problems and occasionally *emphysemia,* (never *emphysema*).

Patients who suffered from *absers* and who requested a dose of *penicillium*, sometimes asked me to 'rip it out'.

I thought this was a dreadful expression, which almost caused me to shudder.

Of course, "Rip it out, mate," should be interpreted as, "Would you please extract my tooth?" I have already mentioned 'the fat man' who seemed to be famous for 'ripping them out'. Sometimes, when a scruffy young individual asked me to 'rip it out, mate', I would respond with, "I'm terribly sorry, but I don't rip teeth out. I could extract the offending molar for you, or, if you have set your heart on having it *ripped out,* I know a rather fat gentleman who will probably oblige you."

A new patient attended my surgery. He was the recently appointed vicar who had been in the town for a little over a year, and he also had a problem with local words and numbers. It was a little different from the word variations I was getting used to, but I suspect it was the same people. He kept chuckling as he explained what had happened.

He was informed that an elderly man had died, and the family wanted him to conduct the funeral. He had never met any of the family before, but visited the widow and bereaved relations. Amongst other matters discussed, he asked them which hymns they would like sung at the service. They looked rather blank, and so he left a hymn book with the family, and said he would return in a few days to note the hymns and finalise the arrangements.

The vicar returned and had another cup of tea with the widow and two or three of the grown up children. He asked them for their choice of hymns, and they gave him the numbers. I cannot remember the specific details, but he was quite bemused to find that they had chosen a Christmas carol, a wedding hymn, a Harvest Festival hymn, and the National Anthem. He enquired why they had chosen those particular hymns.

"We don't know nothing about hymns and things," said the widow, as the others stared vacantly on. "Or church. We did it by the numbers, you see. Number 417 is because he loved his little home, 41 Town Road, and his lucky number was 7. So,

417. Number 156 is his birthday. My boy Fred came up with that. 15th June. Day 15 of month 6. 156. Clever! My Fred's a bright lad. So I learnt from Fred and did our wedding day. Number 222. 22nd of February. Get it? And for the last one, we took part of the number of his favourite car. Loved that Cortina, he did. ADL 672. So we chose 672. That's how we done it, and I think our Walter would be right chuffed with them. So now you know."

I suggested to the vicar that they might have been suffering from absers, or have taken too much penicillium.

* * *

Some of these patients became my friends over the years, including those who had absers, asked for penicillium, and sang *We Three Kings of Orient Are* at funerals. What I saw was what I got, and there was no pretentiousness. Occasionally I would go to their home to explain a treatment, or on one occasion, simply to visit a patient who was housebound with the latter stages of a malignancy of the tongue that I had diagnosed. I would sit and have a cup of tea with them, and enjoy their hospitality. These days I meet them in the supermarket, or whilst walking across the market place. And occasionally, just occasionally, they tell me, "I've had an abser."

* * *

During my years working with the NHS, we were usually paid on a fee per item basis. As a young dentist, I worked fairly quickly, though I have always enjoyed conversation with patients. I did not treat teeth; I treated *people*. There is a difference! But as the years passed, my energy level waned somewhat. Also during this time, I was getting to know my patients better, and there seemed more to talk about. The result of this was that I carried out less treatment, and talked (and listened) more. These two factors, along with an increasingly bureaucratic NHS, made the system difficult to work with. I was loath to leave the NHS as so many of my patients were on government benefits, and could not afford private treatment. However, many of my patients were reasonably affluent and saw me privately anyway. They too had become my friends over the years. And then suddenly the government cut the amount paid to dentists by around 19%. There was no discussion with us, but a unilateral decision in what I felt was a very Cavalier manner. They brought it into effect with one month's notice, whereas we had to give them three months notice if we wished to cease working for them. I felt I needed to make some difficult decisions about my future. Difficult? - it seemed wrong to stay working under the NHS, but also wrong to leave. My final decision was something of a compromise, retaining my private patients, and continuing to see people on government benefits and children as NHS patients so that they did not have to pay. Other people I had previously treated under the NHS could now see me under private contract, a dental insurance scheme, or be treated by one of my younger associates, who would no doubt have more energy.

I suspect that the same decision, in principle, would have been taken by James Bond at some point in his career. There must come a time in life when Secret Service agents can no longer leap from carriage to carriage along the roofs of railway trains, wrestle to the ground villains with stainless steel teeth, abseil down hundreds of feet of vertical rock, or skydive into enemy territory. And likewise, there came a time when I largely bowed out from working for Her Majesty's National Health Service, and some years later, hung up my drill and retired. I enjoyed my work, I loved my patients (most), and I have fabulous memories of many happy years. Now, in the tenth year of my retirement, I remain fit, reasonably energetic, and wonderfully busy.

PART TWO

HEROES, VILLAINS
and MEMORABLE OTHERS

HEROES

The name is Bond. James Bond. In each of the books, and in every film, 007 was the hero. In dictionaries, we read that a hero is a champion, a winner, a brave man.

As far as I was concerned, the central character in my work setting was the patient. The patient was the focus of attention of dentist, clinical and non-clinical staff, and all the other people involved in the practice. Some of my patients were heroes. They were usually brave, and sometimes successful - but not always one of life's winners in the eyes of the world.

Heroes? They were people whose names we enjoyed seeing on our list for the day. They were people who left us feeling better for their visit. They were people who helped others along life's journey. They were people who made us smile. Let me introduce you to a few.

Hero One.   Hammer!
Hero Two.   Whiffler
Hero Three. The Pickled Premolar
Hero Four.   The Man with the Golden Tooth

Hero One.

Hammer!

Bond - James Bond - did not work in isolation. He had his fellow agents and back-up team in London, but there were others. Wherever he went in the world, we find him lining up with the local agents and anti-espionage personnel. In *You Only Live Twice (1967)*, the liaison is with Richard 'Dikko' Henderson in Japan. Often, it is with Felix Leiter of the CIA. But if Bond had ever come to the Norfolk county town where I practised, the local contact would almost certainly have been Clarke - Phillip Clarke.

* * *

It was late in 1984, and my county practice was in its first year. "If this patient has really done a runner, we will have to send Mike Hammer after him," I said with a degree of resignation.

* * *

It was only a few months since Phillip Clarke had first attended my Norfolk surgery. I was fairly new to the quaint little market town where I now worked five half-days a week, though I had cycled there several times as a teenager. My home had been in the next town, just seven miles away by road, but probably significantly nearer as the crow flew. As a lad, I had decided that the road between the two towns must have been put down 'in olden days' because it seemed to go round every field that presented in that part of rural, agricultural Norfolk, such that even on my Trent Tourer bicycle, I had to cycle, brake, cycle, brake and cycle most of the journey. But that was years ago, of course.

Phillip had stepped into the surgery, stopped, gazed around, and then strode over to me.

"The name's Clarke. Phillip Clarke," he said, shaking me firmly by the hand.

He sat in the chair, and I welcomed him to the practice. He was quite smartly attired in a lounge suit, with formal shirt and tie. He must have been a little over six feet in height, and appeared fit.

I perused the information sheet that he had completed at reception prior to coming through to the surgery. Beside each medical question was a short dash. No ticks. No comments at the end of the section. My mind went back to an episode of the comedy series Hancock's Half Hour, where Tony H was asked to fill in such a questionnaire. He answered that he was perfectly fit, that the answer to all the medical questions was 'No', and looking extremely indignant, added, "*and especially that one there!*" Hoots of laughter (at Hancock - not Mr. Clarke). My eye moved down to the section called 'personal', (as though one's medical history and present state of health was *not* personal!)

Male, Married, C of E, and...

'Private detective' had been written beside the question, 'Occupation?'

Mr. Clarke was gazing straight ahead, but I suspect he was actually aware of my every move.

"I see you're a private detective," I ventured, by way of conversation.

"Certainly am," he replied.

"That is absolutely fascinating," I said. I explained that I had now been in practice for a little over fifteen years, and had never had a private detective as a patient before. In fact, I had never knowingly ever *met* a private detective. I enquired what sort of work he undertook.

"Murder, theft, blackmail, and crime of any sort," he explained. "More often than not it's a lady who's suspicious about her husband being out too many evenings, or a husband suspicious of his wife playing too much Bingo. So a lot of the work is surveillance and then reporting back. I have to merge into the shadows, and occasionally adopt a disguise."

"What an exciting life!" I exclaimed.

But time was short, and I needed to get on with his dental examination. He had taken good care of his teeth, and needed little doing, so I referred him to our dental hygienist for a routine appointment, and suggested he return in six months.

"And if I can be of any service to you at any time, don't hesitate to get in touch," he said, handing me his card.

'Phillip Clarke, Private Detective'

Back home at my cottage, my wife and I would talk about our respective day's work, hers on reception and mine in the surgery.

I asked what her impression had been of Phillip Clarke.

"Hammer," she said. "Mike Hammer. He has to be."

"I think you're right," I added. "To begin with, I thought he was Bond. James Bond. But he's certainly more of a Hammer. Mike Hammer. More mature in years than Bond, and he wears the raincoat."

I have had a love/hate relationship with television most of my life. As a child, there was no such thing as television, and I can remember my mother having Housewife's Choice (mainly Perry Como, it seemed) on the wireless in the kitchen while she worked, and Wimbledon for one solid fortnight a year in the summer. Both parents listened to football and cricket, and I listened to 'Journey into Space' starring Andrew Faulds. My sister - I think she played with dolls most of the time. Girls do.

And then father came home from work one evening looking really pleased with himself. About three days later, a Bush twelve inch black and white television was delivered. Our lives were never the same after that, with the whole family now sitting in front of the tiny screen watching hours of Grandstand on Saturday afternoons, and on week nights, early soaps such as The Grove Family, and The Appleyards, not to mention Rawhide and the like.

Years later, as a young dentist, I decided that television had caused me to waste too much time, and so we did not have one. As a result, I missed the first moon landing, and other events and programmes that I would have enjoyed immensely. But by the time I settled into the delightful little rose-coloured cottage in the small village that was just ten minutes drive from my country surgery, I was watching the silver screen most nights. Hence, Mike Hammer.

Mickey Spillane was an American writer of detective tales, and his signature, iconic character was the hard-boiled private eye, Mike Hammer. A series of Mike Hammer was running on television each week, and we never missed it. So when Phillip Clarke presented as a private detective, he just had to be our 'Hammer'.

* * *

A month or two later, a rather different character appeared in the surgery. Rick Muccino was the proprietor of a public house with restaurant in a small village, just three miles out of town. The White Hart was situated down a lane, about two hundred yards from the main Norwich road, and was just visible as we drove towards the city.

Rick Muccino was a smart dresser and a smooth talker. He had masterminded the success of The White Hart and people were travelling from well outside the area in order to indulge themselves in the exquisite culinary delights that were becoming the talk of the county. He told me so. His menu was extensive and his chef had worked in leading hotels in the capital. He told me so. But with his devotion to the gourmet-loving clientele that had been building up over the past two years or so since taking over the establishment, he had rather neglected his teeth. As a result, two had been extracted at another practice in the region, to which he did not wish to return. But now there was a gap, just visible when he smiled. Could I please help him?

With implants yet to be developed, there were the options of gap, plastic denture, metal denture or bridge. A bridge was by far the best, and most expensive, choice, and Rick Muccino was now a rising star within his profession, and his smile was a valued asset. I explained what treatment was involved, and gave a detailed itemised costing. Back in 1984, £600 was probably equivalent to around £2000 at the time of writing (2016). The cost? £600 was no problem to a gentleman of Mr. Muccino's standing.

Around a month later the treatment was complete, and after flashing his new smile at me, Rick said I should bring my wife out to his restaurant one evening, where we would be treated like royalty.

Reception sent Rick an account for £600 at the end of the month, but it was not paid. A second account was sent the following month, with the same result, and a third and final account one month later. Shortly after that, we were driving into the city one evening, and I decided to call in at The White Hart to see if there was a problem with the treatment I had provided for Rick Muccino. I thought that I might also book in for the promised dinner.

There were no curtains at the windows, and the door was locked. Spiders' webs had remained undamaged around the doorframe for quite some time, and the menu, just visible through a glass frame that was almost opaque with accumulated dust, was three months out of date. Across the lane a cottage window creaked open.

"You looking for Muccino?" called a voice. "Well, he's gone. And if he owes you money, hard luck, cos' nobody knows where."

£600 was a lot of money to me in those days, with a wife, four beautiful daughters, a mortgage, and a thousand other expenses. But what could I do?

"Hammer is what you can do," said my wife. "If anyone can track down the foul felon, Hammer is the man."

And so, on returning home that evening, I searched for the little business card I had been handed around four months previously, and decided to engage the services of a private detective.

* * *

"I'm your man," said my new friend Phillip. "Clarke's the name. Phillip Clarke. Leave it to me." And having noted down the details of the treacherous Muccino, he swung round on his heel and marched out of the surgery.

"See you've had the bailiff in," said my next patient, as he sat in my chair removing half his mouth and depositing it in a glass beaker that my nurse had extended towards him. "Not paid your bills, have you!" he added with a slimy wet chuckle.

"Bailiff?" I asked

"Your last patient," said the patient, and went on to explain. "He's the local bailiff. Not paid your bill, and he's the one they send round. Look at the front of his reinforced boots. Flattened they are, from kicking doors in. And I bet his front teeth aren't his own. Or maybe he wears a gum shield when he's at work."

So that was Phillip's main line of work. And what chance did I stand of him tracing a slippery character like Muccino and recovering the money he owed me? Maybe he could kick doors in and withstand a few punches to the upper incisors, but when a villain vanished into thin air...

* * *

Two days later, my wife opened the surgery door between patients and with an excited grin, said, "Hammer's back. He wants to see you."

"Clarke's your man. Phillip Clarke," said the chap himself as he entered the surgery. He had a twinkle in his eye, as he announced his coup.

"Traced your man, sir. He's currently enjoying the high life with your £600 and several thousand more withheld from other business people in this area. Anyway, that's their problem. Should have come to me like you did. But he'll be arriving at his new restaurant just outside Portsmouth at the end of this week. And when he does, Justin Defreine, as he will be known at his new establishment, will find a bill waiting for him. I've added a few words of my own to the account, and I'll be surprised if it's not settled by the end of next week."

Phillip, my almost-best friend, smiled at me in a knowing way - and was gone.

Towards the end of the following week, I received a cheque for £600 settling Rick Muccino's account.

And after that, on those very few occasions when I had a problem with an unpaid account, my wife would say, "Hammer."

And I would look at her and say, "Hammer."

And the man with the reinforced boots and raincoat would collect a few details, slip out of the surgery, merge with the shadows, and vanish into the night.

Hero Two.

Whiffler!

Jaws was not his real name, but it described him absolutely. The late Richard Kiel stood seven feet three inches high, and had metal teeth fitted in order to play the vicious character in two of the Bond films – *The Spy Who Loved Me (1977)* and *Moonraker (1979)*. The late Hervé Jean-Pierre Villechaize, who played *Nick Nack* in the film *The Man With The Golden Gun (1974)*, was three foot and one inch high. As a diminutive servant and general dog's body, the name *Nick Nack* described him beautifully. At school, almost everyone had a nickname. I was *Snowball*. It was my hair, you see. I felt sorry for *Bog Rat!* But - who was *Whiffler*?

* * *

"Hey, that article in the newspaper is about *our* surgery!" said my receptionist.

For most of my life I have been a *Daily Telegraph* man; except on Sunday, that is, when I have taken the *Sunday Telegraph*. Most of us become familiar with a particular newspaper, and naturally different people like different papers. I think I was quite young when I picked up my paternal grandfather's *Daily Telegraph*, and that was my introduction. My parents always read the *Daily Mail*, which I scanned through each day during my teenage years; *and* it was the *Mail* where I started wrestling with cryptic crosswords. Thank you *Daily Mail*. But on Sundays, *The People* and the *Sunday*

Express were delivered, and I must confess that the former had me spellbound at times. Did people really get up to such things?

As a dentist, there were times when I had real problems with the *Daily Mail*. It had a tendency towards sensationalism, which appeals to a certain type of reader and sells plenty of newspapers. But when I started reading that root treating teeth can lead to strokes and heart attacks, and that root-filled teeth, and all teeth that have, or have had, an abscess, should be extracted, I started doubting what I read in other articles too. And then, when this aficionado of Indian food read that eating curry can cause gum disease... which confirmed me as a reader of the *Daily* and *Sunday Telegraphs*.

Daphne, my receptionist looked up from her *Eastern Daily Press*, the country's best selling regional newspaper.

"It *must* be our practice that I'm reading about in here," she said. "Take it and have a look. Surely no-one else has an aerial photograph of Norwich city centre on their surgery ceiling."

I took the paper, known locally as the EDP, and started reading. 'As I lay back in my dentist's chair, trying to relax, I gazed up at the aerial photograph of Norwich city centre that was fixed to the ceiling directly overhead. I started planning a route...'

The article was written by 'Whiffler' - but who was Whiffler? He was obviously fascinated with the aerial photograph on my surgery ceiling. And not only he!

When I bought the practice in 1973, the ceilings were bare. Well, most people have bare ceilings. I had been in practice for five years, working in Dorset in another man's practice. We had been given advice back at dental school, "Once you're qualified, wait awhile before setting up your own practice. Go and make your mistakes on somebody else's patients first, and then, when you can do it properly, start your own practice - and be careful who you take on to work on *your* patients!" I bought the Norwich practice in November 1973, and opened for business January 1974. The previous dentist, Andrew Trevelyan, was hugely respected within the profession, and in fact had been working there for twenty years. During that time, dentistry had changed, and I wanted to stamp my own personality on the practice. One idea was to do something creative with the ceilings. Many surgeries still had the ancient cast-iron upright dental chairs, which meant that the patient stared straight ahead. But new chairs, which tipped back almost horizontally, were slowly being introduced. These chairs meant that the dentist could now sit down to work, and it was said in our journals that this would be the end of dentists having back trouble and varicose veins, both of which occurred in over fifty percent of the profession. It did - dentists no longer had such a high incidence of backache and varicose veins, but instead developed quite serious neck problems from craning over the patient from the sitting position.

So the patient now gazed up, and I thought it would be novel to give them something to look at. I sought advice from a designer, who suggested an aerial photograph of Norwich. In fact, there was a second downstairs room, which I was going to use as another surgery, for an associate dentist (if I could find one), and so we searched for a photograph for each. My designer friend located some four-inch square negatives of the centre of the city taken by the Royal Air Force, and two of them were 'blown up' to four-foot square prints and mounted on wood. The definition of the originals, from many years previously, must have been amazing. Each was fixed to a surgery ceiling. Some of the comments were fascinating, and some were amusing.

"Now let me see," said an architect patient, after I had tipped the chair back. "I should be able to date that photograph by the extensions on certain buildings. Do you see the building on the left side of St. Giles Street, about a third of the way down... See. Now that wasn't there until 1959. But we need more clues..."

"Hey, that bus shouldn't be going along there. That's a number thirty-five, that is. Cor, that must be at least ten years ago. I'm a bus driver, you see, and I know," said another.

"Look mate - the old toilets by the market are still there. They've moved them now. Got new ones we have. That dates it," said a man in a shabby raincoat.

But who was Whiffler? I looked the word up in an encyclopaedia, and apparently the whiffler was a man who went ahead of a procession and cleared the way by waving a javelin. That was in the sixteenth century. And it could also refer to a man who 'whiffled', which apparently meant shifting around in the course of an argument. So there was not much of a clue there.

However, later that week, the mystery was cleared up, when a patient called John Kett phoned the practice to say that he hoped it was alright using my surgery photographs to illustrate his feature in the EDP. Apparently he had a weekly column, and amongst other things, enjoyed writing in the Norfolk dialect.

Over the following two or three decades, I looked forward to John Kett's visits to my surgery, originally in Norwich, and later at my country practice, which was nearer his home. What a great Norfolk name! Robert Kett had led a peasant's rebellion in Norfolk in the sixteenth century. He was not a peasant himself, but when targeted by the rebels, joined and led them as he was sympathetic to their cause. With an army of sixteen thousand he defeated the army led by the Marquess of Northampton, though he was later defeated and hanged from the walls of Norwich castle.

John Kett was headmaster of a school around ten miles from Norwich. His account of one of his early experiences had me doubled up laughing, and is a story I continue to relate at dinner parties. Different parts of the country have surnames which are almost exclusive to that particular region, and Norfolk is no exception. One surname which can be found quite extensively in certain parts of the county is Tortice. Having arrived at the school to take up his duties as headmaster, John Kett attended a Parent-Teacher Association meeting. He was introduced to numerous parents of pupils at the school, including a Mrs. Tortice. This was a new name to John, and he thought it most unusual. He wondered if it might be spelt t-o-r-t-o-i-s-e but on looking through the school records, realised it was t-o-r-t-i-c-e. Later that week, he was strolling through the village of Cawston where the school was situated, when round the corner ahead of him walked the lady with the unusual name. She smiled at him as she approached, and John suddenly found his mind had gone completely blank. She was barely ten yards away and he was really struggling now. Suddenly his mind seemed to clear, and in response to, "Good afternoon, Mr. Kett" from the parent, the headmaster replied, "And good afternoon to you too, Mrs. Hedgehog." Thirty seconds later he stopped dead in his tracks and froze. *Not* Hedgehog - Tortice.

John would tell me of his love affair with Iceland. He and his wife Mary would frequently visit the country, and enthuse over the pastel shades of colour due to the light there. Some years later I was to go there for myself and check it out. It was true, of course. John and Mary were committed Christians, and he was a lay reader in the Church of England. We discovered that his son had been at school with me (though several years lower), and he and his family became patients. One year, David Kett and I went together to our Old Boys dinner.

When John retired from being headmaster at Cawston school, he was cheered by the pupils (including some Tortices) and given a bicycle. He continued to write in the EDP, and published a number of books written in the Norfolk dialect, and a further book as a tribute to his wife Mary after she died.

John Kett, Whiffler, headmaster, storyteller, journalist and author, who died at the age of ninety-three just before Christmas 2010. John - you were an inspiration!

Hero Three.

The Pickled Premolar!

'A medium vodka dry Martini, with a slice of lemon peel. Russian or Polish vodka. Shaken, not stirred,' was the full description of how Bond usually ordered a drink. He first uttered those words in the novel, *Doctor No*. In January 2016, Wendy and I took a succession of funicular railways and cable cars to reach Blofeld's mountain lair featured in *On Her Majesty's Secret Service (1969)*. At over 9,700 feet, and perched on the summit of the Schilthorn in the Swiss Alps, is the James Bond restaurant. We ordered, and enjoyed, a vodka Martini, shaken not stirred.

But Bond consumed other alcoholic drinks. Often. In large doses. Dom Pérignon 1953 was his preferred champagne. During a scene in *A View To A Kill (1985)*, where Bond spends an evening having dinner with Stacey Sutton (Tanya Roberts), I have always been fascinated that, despite there being three empty wine bottles on the table, Bond is super-athletic in seeing off a gang of assassins. Most people would be completely pickled.

Which leads me to the story of the pickled premolar, as my friend Peter described it. But I thought that it was actually the *patient* that was pickled. What do you think?

* * *

It was Christmas Day, the turkey with all the trimmings had been carved into generous portions, laying alongside equally humongous piles of vegetables - with maybe just the odd sprout for the children. After sploshing more than ample quantities of fine red wine into more than ample wine glasses, Peter stood to his feet at the head of the table.

"Wait!" he said, smiling broadly and training his eyes on the children. "Before *anyone* starts, I am going to propose a toast. Please be upstanding with me in toasting - 'My dentist, Barrie Lawrence, without whom I would be unable to enjoy my turkey today.'"

* * *

Peter first came to my city practice in the late 1970s. He had been suffering from intermittent chronic toothache for some months. Now, the intermittent had gone, and the continuous had set in, and the chronic gnawing ache had evolved into sharp acute pain.

He was unable even to drive his car. It was not primarily his toothache, but the medication he had taken for it, from a bottle emanating from a Scottish distillery. To use Peter's own words, he had 'pickled' the tooth.

His wife helped him out of the car and guided him to the front door of the practice. They arrived at reception, and Peter propped himself up on the counter while Gillian explained.

"My husband has had toothache for several months, and it has just got worse and worse. Now he can't even drive, because he's pickled it. Please can Mr. Lawrence have a look at the tooth for him?"

And so Peter was helped up the stairs of my city practice, and as soon as I had opportunity, I invited him into the surgery. He gave me a strange smile and lurched to the chair, supported by his wife and my nurse. I asked if I could have a look at the tooth, and he leant back and opened his mouth.

Pow - I felt just a little giddy myself as fumes heavy with Scotch whisky ascended from the pickled premolar. It was decayed. It was fractured. It had abscessed. And it needed a lot of treatment. But to make life more tolerable for Peter, I simply prescribed antibiotic tablets and suggested a further appointment.

His wife explained to me that Peter had only come to my surgery because I carried out intravenous anaesthetics ('needle in the arm' to knock the patient out). We arranged a number of appointments, all under I.V., and by Christmas, Peter had a stable pain-free dentition. And so, with the turkey carved and waiting on their plates, his family was upstanding and drank my health.

* * *

All that was many years ago, but we have stayed in touch, even though I am now retired. Peter is a carpenter, and the most scholarly carpenter I know. He is knowledgeable about classical music, and especially Elgar, Mozart and Wagner. He is a formidable opponent at golf - and so friendly with it. But that's Peter - always smiling, always good-humoured, and someone who always leaves you feeling better for having spent time chatting with him.

And so I raise my glass to Peter, and wish him good health and prosperity!

Hero Four.

The Man with the Golden Tooth

The word *gold* appears twice in the titles of James Bond books by Ian Fleming, namely *Goldfinger* and *The Man with the Golden Gun*, and also in the film *Goldeneye (1995)*, not based on a book by Fleming. *Goldeneye* is one of my favourite non-Fleming Bond films. There is something attractive about gold, not least its perceived intrinsic value and stability, such that when world economies start to wobble, gold is viewed by many as a safe haven for their wealth.

Gold has other valuable properties, which have resulted in it being used for restoring teeth; not for centuries, but for millennia. The ancient Egyptians replaced teeth using gold wires and plates around 2000 B.C., which is four thousand years ago. The gold is still intact today, as is that used by the Mayans in Central America more recently, at around 800 A.D. It is very workable, being malleable (one can beat it into shape) and ductile (one can 'draw it out' into shape), both properties useful to ancient civilisations. Today, it is heated until molten, and cast.

But it is expensive, and not everyone can afford to have a vintage Rolls Royce made of solid gold, as Goldfinger did for his smuggling operations. Likewise, the ex-circus performer Scaramanga, with his golden gun. And then there was my patient and friend, Denis. Let me tell you about him.

* * *

"Just pull it out and stick me a gold one there," said Denis Hewson. He was not the first, and he would not be the last. Quite a number of people want to be 'the man with the golden tooth.'

* * *

The first time I met Denis, he greeted me like an old friend. I thought he must have known me. Maybe he did, but I could not recall having seen him before.

With a wide, toothy grin, he shook me by the hand and greeted me with, "Hello Barrie. How are you doing, mate?"

Everybody loved Denis. He was friendly, kind, encouraging, and with a great sense of humour. He looked as though he purchased his clothes from the Salvation Army charity shop - but I'm sure he could have bought me out several times over.

Denis sat in my chair, and asked me to have a look round and tell him what needed doing. His teeth looked good, and likewise his gums and the partial denture at the top.

"I'll be back," he said with that wide smile. "And if you haven't been to my new restaurant at The Wheatsheaf, do come and give us a try. Special deal for you."

The Wheatsheaf? I had passed it a thousand times, but did not know there was a restaurant there. Surely it was a Bed and Breakfast. I mentioned this to a chap in our village who knew everything and everyone. Denis lived in the village, but I thought he ran the garage.

"Denis? The Wheatsheaf? Yes, he's probably running it as a restaurant," said Chris. "He's been running the service station for some years, but I think the Browns have bought it from him. Not sure. You never can be with Denis. Nice bloke, though. He's like King Midas - everything he touches turns to gold."

And eventually his teeth started to as well.

So he had sold the service station, and was running The Wheatsheaf. Christmas was approaching, and I always took my in-laws out for a Christmas dinner a week or two before the actual day. I telephoned The Wheatsheaf.

"Could I book six of us in for a Christmas dinner early in December please?" I asked the lady who answered the telephone. The arrangements were made. I asked the lady on the phone to let Denis Hewson know that I had booked in. She giggled.

"Certainly will," said Hannah. "He's a very good friend of mine, is Denis." More giggling.

* * *

Ours was the only table occupied that evening, but Denis and Hannah prepared us a fine meal. They appeared to be doing all the work themselves, and as well as cooking and waiting at the table, would periodically stick their heads round the door from the kitchen and together, give us huge smiles. The Wheatsheaf was now a hotel, but there did not seem to be anybody staying there.

At the end of the evening, Denis and Hannah came to the door of the hotel and shook our hands. They gave us the widest of smiles.

* * *

When he was next at the surgery for his six-monthly examination, I asked Denis how The Wheatsheaf was doing. He pulled a face and shook his head.

"Hannah has gone. Just left, and I don't know where. And she's taken ten thousand pounds that belongs to *me*. I've had enough. I'm selling up. I'm going to have a garden centre instead. I'll run it with my wife, and we'll move our museum and shops there as well." There was not so much as the hint of a smile.

Museum? Apparently, during the war, an American bomber had taken off from the airbase two miles outside the village, clipped a tree half a mile away, and crashed in flames on our village common. Denis and a few others had braved the fire to rescue the crew, and now had a museum commemorating the event.

Shops? Bric a Brac, and an extensive assortment of anything and everything probably describes them best.

* * *

"Just pull it out and stick me a gold one there," said Denis after I had examined his upper left canine, from which an enormous filling had fallen out.

I could have crowned it. Maybe, but as there was a significant chance of it failing, and as most of Denis' top teeth were replaced by a denture anyway, he asked me to remove it.

"But I want a gold one in its place. Can you do that?" he asked with that big grin that had returned.

I explained that instead of colour matching, and replacing the natural tooth with a denture tooth that looked like it, I could instruct the technicians to use a gold tooth.

"But it's a canine, Denis. It's almost at the forefront of your smile. Everybody will see it," I warned.

"Just what I want," was the grinning reply. "I shall be famous around these parts. I'll be the man with the golden tooth!"

And within a week, Denis was indeed just that. He thanked me profusely, and questioned the fee as it seemed quite low, he said. I explained that the tooth was hollow, and now housed acrylic from the denture that would help keep it in place "Not solid, but no-one would know. Best hollow, and costs less too," I added.

And whenever I went to the garden centre, where the museum and shops are still housed, and where he created a dirt track for speedway riders next door ("used to be a rider myself once," he said with sparkly smile), he would grin broadly, and say, "The man with the golden tooth."

And people in the village would ask one another whether they had seen Denis recently. And they would add, "He calls himself, 'The man with the golden tooth.'

RIP Denis Hewson (not his real name of course) - you are greatly missed around our village and area. Entrepreneur. Garage proprietor. Hotelier. Proprietor of garden centre and shops. Everybody's friend. Man with the golden tooth!

VILLAINS

Blofeld was a villain. So was Le Chiffre, Mr. Big, Sir Hugo Drax, and countless others. I looked up the definition of a villain in some dictionaries. There are many words there that describe such a person, but I have finally gone for simplicity; a villain is a person who does bad things.

If we are honest, there are times when most of us have done bad things. And then psychology comes into play, suggesting that if we have done more good than bad, we are OK really; or we are convinced that many other people have done worse. Maybe so, but my Bible tells me clearly that even 'good' people will not get into heaven. No-one is good enough, except Jesus, and so only *forgiven* people will enter heaven.

During my years in practice, I saw people who repeatedly did bad things. Some were charming, and some were certainly not. They cheated. They lied. And they never changed. They were villains. Here come two, plus a house-full - watch out!

Villain One.   **A Burger Too Far**

Villain Two.   **Dick Jones**

Villain(s) Three.   **The Blue House**

Villain One.

A Burger Too Far

Ernst Stavro Blofeld was Bond's arch enemy. He is portrayed in different ways by a variety of actors who played the part. One thing that all the real villains seem to have in common, is being hospitable to 007, and he is invariably sitting at table with them. Blofeld is one, and likewise Dr. No, Kamal Khan, Scaramanga, and a number of others. Klaus Maria Brandauer plays Maximillian Largo in *Never Say Never Again (1983)*. He is villainous, deadly, probably psychotic, and - totally charming. He entertained Bond on his yacht, and I'm sure he was the perfect host at dinner. He reminds me of a patient.

* * *

André was an award-winning restaurateur, but calling in at McDonalds one evening was 'a burger too far'. He lost absolutely everything.

André had come to Norfolk as a young man, and excelled at managing public houses. He enjoyed chatting with the local people, and they found his charm magnetic. He was successful. He fell in love with Di, and she with him. They married, and she joined him in his work.

* * *

I was unaware that a local celebrity had walked into my surgery. André Lefever was smartly dressed, and would probably be described as 'cool' by people a generation or more younger than me. He was charming, polite, and well spoken but not posh.

"I've heard all about you," he said. 'You're the man to come to round here. By the way, have I seen you at The Nelson yet? Well worth a visit – *my* guest."

I had heard vaguely of The Nelson, which was situated out in the back of beyond for those who could navigate the Norfolk lanes that led there. It had been a quiet little haven for the agricultural community who had patronised it for generations - until André and Di arrived. They had seen the potential, and within a year it was humming with people. It was heavily beamed, with an ambience of rural romance. Roaring log-fires and an extensive menu not only brought in successful businessmen and holidaymakers from the region and beyond, but also triggered a series of features in upmarket glossy magazines. André was becoming famous within the county - and Di was working tirelessly in the kitchens.

"Whatever is needed," said André, leaning back in the chair and winking at my nurse. "It's been a while since I came to one of these places, but you tell me what needs doing. As many appointments as it takes - might even enjoy coming." Another wink at the nurse. "Cost no problem. Cash - straight into your pocket!"

André did indeed need a modest amount of treatment, and attended regularly until his dentition was back in order. I preferred patients to pay reception rather than me personally, and André always paid on the way out. Cash. Cash that had probably gone 'straight into *his* pocket'.

"Did you see André on television last night?" asked my nurse. "He is a lovely man - absolutely charming. Told me he'd buy me a drink at his restaurant one evening if I'd like to go there. Lovely man."

I enquired why André had been on television the previous night, and was informed that it was the local news programme, and it was to do with his pies.

"His pies?" I exclaimed. "What's so special about André's pies?"

"Best in the county," I was informed. "He said he was going in for a national competition. Could be the best in the country soon."

A few weeks later Di came in. André might have been a smooth charmer heralding from some urban metropolis, but Di was Norfolk. While André gyrated from table to table in the evenings, shaking hands with those honoured to meet the man himself, Di just got on with the cooking. Di supervised the kitchen, trained up assistant chefs, and it was Di who made the pies.

"Have you seen us on television?" she asked. I replied that I had certainly heard all about the news coverage of their award winning pies, and Di brought out a folded newspaper article on the award ceremony, with a photograph of the two of them holding up a pie, whilst another local celebrity displayed a large certificate that was being presented to them.

"It's hard work in those kitchens. Hot too," said Di. "And André is off on another holiday. Again. Ireland this time, fishing, and then he comes back for two weeks before going off to Scandinavia. He has worked so hard in the past, and deserves his holidays. I just wish we could go together. But I'll get two weeks in the Mediterranean sun when he gets back. That'll do me."

The restaurant went from strength to strength, and tables had to be booked well in advance. The walls were clad with award certificates, and André was fêted as one of Norfolk's great success stories. Well done André, and well done the chef!

* * *

It was two or three years since the pie awards had started being chalked up, and André was spending more and more time out celebrating with friends (he now had a lot of friends) or holidaying abroad. Di was still working long hours in the kitchens, and quietly proud of her husband's achievements.

André had driven into the city for a drink with friends, and at the end of the evening got behind the wheel to drive himself back to The Nelson. But beer can make a man hungry, and beer was what André had been drinking. And wine. Also, a few spirits to round off the evening.

Driving towards home took him round the ring road, when hunger suddenly struck. Almost immediately, some golden arches came into view. Swinging into the car park was perhaps a mistake, as walking in anything resembling a straight line was near impossible by now. The Drive Thru' might have been safer, but then again, could André have *driven* in a straight line?

Bumping into a table or two on his way, André approached the counter and ordered a Big Mac meal. The staff were amused, but when a young lass realised he was going to *drive* away, she became alarmed.

"He could kill someone. Easily," she said to her colleagues.

"Guess you're right," said the manager, as André stumbled towards the door, leaving a trail of fries in his wake. "I'll phone the police."

* * *

AWARD WINNING RESTAURATEUR ARRESTED IN McDONALDS CAR PARK, was the headline in a respectable local newspaper. *CELEBRITY CHEF HAS HAD HIS CHIPS* ran another less prestigious rag.

And whereas André had cruised to great heights over just a few years, he suddenly nose-dived into obscurity in a matter of weeks. He pleaded guilty to drunken driving, at more than three times over the legal limit. He was disqualified from driving. He was fined heavily, but could not pay. Bankruptcy quickly followed and, whilst following hard on the drink-driving conviction, was in fact due to too much holiday, not enough time at work, and too much gambling. And then he vanished. Di continued working in the kitchens under the new management, but as divorce proceeded, moved on to other catering appointments where she was not known as the celebrity pie maker.

* * *

And then, one Sunday she came into our church in the market town where I had treated her and André at my surgery years earlier. Well, I thought it was her, though the passing of time does tend to change us.

"Is it Di?" I enquired.

"Mr. Lawrence!" she replied. "I didn't know you came here."

I enquired why she had come to our service that morning, and she told me that since leaving The Nelson, life had not been the happy adventure she had once experienced. Work was not plentiful, and pennies were few. She lived by herself, and had come along that morning to see 'what went on'.

My wife and I were lunching at home by ourselves, and Di had nothing planned - so she came back with us. After roast pork (first class, thanks to Wendy, but gaining no official awards), we sat by our log fire and enjoyed a glass of wine after which we all dozed off for a while!

Di came along to our church quite often, and usually came back for lunch and a glass of wine by the log fire. Life in the fast lane had led to fame and fortune. But even for those who are able to retain it, there is not the depth of fulfillment and lasting satisfaction that comes from a real relationship with the God we read of in the Bible, and who we can truly come to know through the Lord Jesus Christ. I know. It happened to me.

And Di? One day she was gone. We emailed, and she told me she had moved to a coastal town in North Norfolk where she had a small flat, and had been offered part-time work. Wendy and I still feel sad for Di. And I feel sad for André too, the celebrity charmer, and award winning pie man who simply went 'a burger too far'!

Villain Two.

Dick Jones

Auric Goldfinger was quite ruthless. He was totally dedicated to selfish personal gain. He was a bully. His name was pretentious. He would never have gone under the name of Dick Jones

* * *

"My name is Richard Harrison Barrington-Jones - and I want you to take me on as your patient. I am not going back to that other ******* ****."

I was at a cocktail party to celebrate the opening of a new insurance office in the town. The company had been extremely helpful in assisting me set up my new practice locally. Chris, the branch manager and his wife had been patients at my city practice for several years, and when I told them I was hoping to start a branch practice in the town where they lived, they were enthusiastic. My main problem was raising the capital needed to buy the property in which to house the practice. Eventually it was a joint effort with the local bank providing a loan and the insurers helping me to set up the necessary security.

The practice had taken off from day one, and though I was only working there half-days (but every day), I was rushed off my feet as patients piled in. Chris and his wife were so helpful, recommending people to the practice, as well as providing free weekday accommodation for my nurse/receptionist, who lived twelve miles away and had no transport of her own.

So we were at the cocktail party, and Chris was his usual bundle of energy, gyrating around the crowded office with bottles and glasses, ricocheting from person to person whilst engaging in animated conversation with guests representing so many of the local traders and significant businesses. A rather stout middle-aged gentleman, dressed in a grey suit that had probably fitted well before the waistline expanded, kept looking towards me and was clearly moving in my direction. His alcohol-fuelled conversation was loud, and he spoke with a posh accent. Before long he was at my side, breathing intoxicating fumes over me, sweating profusely and tapping me clumsily on the arm in order to gain my attention. As if I had not noticed him already!

"You the new dentist, old boy?"

"Certainly am," I replied. "Been working down the road a few months, and just love this town and the people."

"Well, I've been here a few years now, and some of the local people are absolute *******," he said, using language that took me back to the playground at my primary school.

"I'm surprised," I replied. This little town had been like a refuge for me when my domestic situation had disintegrated a few years earlier, and a local couple had welcomed me as part of their family at that time. They had been a Godsend to me, in the true sense of the word.

"Well, I've heard that you're OK," he said with a sneer. "By the way, my name is Richard Harrison Barrington-Jones - and I want you to take me on as your patient. I am not going back to that other ******* ****."

I almost gasped. Maybe I had led a rather sheltered life, but I had not heard such obscenities since leaving school, and only the roughest of the rough would use such expressions then.

Rather reluctantly I told him that he could phone the surgery and make an appointment to see me anytime. But it took him a year or more, by which time I was incredibly busy and had taken on a younger dentist to help me. So John got him!

* * *

"I see you were talking to Dick Jones the other evening," said Harry Pascoe, a fairly new patient, as he entered the surgery and walked towards the chair.

"Dick Jones?" I asked. "I don't recall meeting anyone called Dick Jones. Where did you see me."

"Across the room at the cocktail party in Red Lion Street," was the reply. "Dick Jones. Big chap. Stomach. Loud voice."

"Dick Jones? I think you mean Richard Harrison Barrington-Jones," I replied. "Yes, I had not met him before and he came over and introduced himself."

"Well, be careful of him," said Harry. "Be careful with... er... Mr. Barrington-Jones."

"Are you telling me his name is not Barrington-Jones?" I asked Harry Pascoe. "And why should I be careful?"

"Well firstly, I knew that man when we were at school together, and at that time his name was Dick Jones," confided my patient, "and secondly, I heard that his last dentist accompanied him to a cash machine in order to receive payment before he would treat him. Unprofessional - but prudent, in my opinion."

And little by little, different patients, friends and acquaintances, by way of conversation, gave me a fuller picture of... er... Mr. Barrington-Jones.

"He started out helping the chef at the Rose and Crown. He was young Dick Jones in those days," said one.

"He got the sack from the Rose and Crown and vanished. Then a year or two later *Richard* Jones was assistant chef at The Red Lion. There was some trouble, and suddenly he was gone," confided another. And there was more.

"I heard he had been working at The Red Lion, and then I saw him at The Lord Nelson. Apparently he was landlord there, and called Richard *Harrison* Jones, so I heard, and then he was gone. Lots of people said he owed them money."

"I used to work for him at The Lord Nelson. The menu said 'lashings of mushrooms' but he said we were to put no more than three on a plate. And he swore at us, lots he did,"

"You know that rather expensive food shop in town? That was him. He was Richard Harrison *Barrington*-Jones by that time, but it closed suddenly. He had lots of debts."

* * *

A few years had passed and a new restaurant had opened a few miles out of town. It had features on it in one of the local newspapers and a glossy magazine that covered the area. Real gourmet stuff. Amazing menu. Celebrity chef. Atmospheric. Rural charm.

Wendy and I went there for a drink one evening after taking a walk through the beautiful north Norfolk countryside. It was early autumn, and a deep plummy sun was grazing the horizon as we entered the bar area of the recently opened restaurant.

"A glass of red wine please, and an orange juice and lemonade for the driver - me!"

A portly gentleman strode into the room and stepped behind the bar.

"Good evening sir," he greeted the gentleman to my right, who had booked a table and was ordering preprandial aperitifs. "I believe I saw you here with Lord Aston last night." (I have changed the name of the titled gentleman).

"Lord Aston? Good gracious, No. I don't know Lord Aston - or any other lords, for that matter," stammered the gentleman.

"So sorry. I was sure it was you that was here with his lordship last night. Anyway, Richard Harrison Barrington-Jones. So pleased to meet you, and I trust that you will enjoy your evening here with us."

As Dick Jones, aka Richard Jones, aka Richard Harrison Barrington-Jones walked back through to the restaurant, the gentleman on my right turned to his wife and companions and said, "Lord Aston comes here. He was here last night. We are at a truly upmarket establishment this evening. Expect it will cost a packet, but it must be worth it - Lord Aston comes here."

The party of four were called and shown through to their table.

"Hey, Mr. Lawrence. Fancy seeing you here." It was Harry Pascoe, sitting in an alcove with his wife, and enjoying a pint. "This is my local. Sort of. Not like it used to be. But I've been coming for years, you see. Under new management now - though I preferred the old. Every evening - 'I believe I saw you here with Lord Aston last night.' Prepares them for the charges. And then, maybe one evening Lord Aston will come in and overhear. What fun. Hope I'm here if it happens."

* * *

Now I'm retired - and so is he. Or is he? Suddenly, he was gone. A new couple had taken over the... well, I'm not going to name the place. But I hear they are doing well. I think Wendy and I might go there one evening, perhaps after a stroll through Lord Aston's estate. And in the meantime, I would not be surprised if I picked up a glossy magazine and found a review of a new sophisticated gourmet restaurant, where proprietor Sir Richard Harrison Barrington-Jones, said, "Our extensive and exquisitely crafted menu of unique gourmet dishes of the highest quality, is enjoyed by our equally unique and exquisite clientele. As I was saying to the Duke of Edinburgh only yesterday evening... "

Villain(s) Three.

The Blue House

"Good morning, Moneypenny," greeted 007 as he breezed through her office, having lobbed his bowler hat onto a coat hook - from outside the open door. He tapped on the door leading to the office of 'M', head of MI5, strode in energetically, and the two of them proceeded to discuss how to save the world from the latest international villain.

SPECTRE, the sinister organisation headed by Blofeld, would sometimes be shown meeting together, and planning vile plots. There were many of them sitting around a huge table, and everyone of them was a ruthless, lethal criminal.

There were times when I could imagine meetings similar to those of SPECTRE taking place in The Blue House.

* * *

"You'll end up in the Blue House!" shouted one of the boys emerging from a fray in the village where I lived as a boy. "That's where you'll end up. The Blue House."

* * *

I suppose it was a sort of Borstal, where young lads who had chalked up sufficient offences were sent to be rehabilitated. No-one really seemed to know too much about the place, but the words *Blue House* were almost whispered, as though we did not want to properly acknowledge that such a place existed.

In Home Office terms of the day, it was a reformatory for the correction of young offenders.

Decades later I opened a dental practice just three miles from the *Blue House*. It had changed its name to the *Oak Tree Academy*, and had been sold to a Scandinavian company who charged the government large sums of money to house and correct delinquent youths. Before long there was a spate of burglaries and arson attacks in the area and, when they were found to be occurring within a two-mile radius of the Oak Tree Academy, security at the place was investigated and found to be woefully inadequate.

One of my associate dentists bought a property approximately one mile from the institution, and would often arrive in the morning with stories of a high police presence in the vicinity of his home, and rumours of escapees being rounded up and taken away in vans.

Occasionally the Academy would telephone my practice and ask for an appointment for one of their charges. Once they had arrived, we would always see them as soon as possible – for the sake of the other patients waiting. "Nice set of wheels yer got outside, mate," said one of the lads as he entered the surgery, and then descended into colourful language to describe the nature of his dental problem.

I returned from a fortnight's holiday one summer, to be greeted with, "You should have been here last week when that *Oak Tree Academy* sent some boys in. One was booked in with toothache, and he brought three of his mates with him. And one kept picking his nose and flicking the bits round the waiting room. It was really horrible, but he looked quite intimidating, and no-one said anything. We tried to get them all out as quickly as possible."

"Was there no-one from the Academy in charge of them?" I asked. "They have always sent one of the staff along with them before."

"That's who it was," said the receptionist. "It was the

member of staff who was picking and flicking his nose around the place. I think he was just showing off to the boys."

Then the Scandinavian company that owned the academy bought property on a Caribbean island, and boys who seriously misbehaved, or who offended frequently, were transferred to the Caribbean. The crime rate in the vicinity of the home increased significantly until all the major delinquents managed to get themselves transferred to the land of sunshine, beaches and bikini-clad ladies. Local residents gave a sigh of relief.

So did my dental associate who lived so close to the institution – until his car went missing one night. What followed was the stuff that comedy films are made of. A policeman arrived and took details of the stolen vehicle, and returned the following day with both good news and bad news. Well, good news for my dentist colleague. The car had been found abandoned in a different county, but another car, of the same make, but of higher specification, had gone missing half a mile distant from it. My friend asked if they had caught the two lads presumed to be the culprits (as they were missing from the academy), but there was no trace of them or the recently stolen car. The following day the missing car was found abandoned like the first one, in a different county. And again, another car, younger and of a higher specification had gone missing in the vicinity. The young villains were eventually apprehended, but not before they had 'traded in' a further two or three cars and helped themselves to newer and more powerful vehicles each time.

It really did seem like a den of thieves, and this opinion appeared to be confirmed when the head of the Scandinavian company that ran the home was arrested in the United States on charges of financial fraud, followed by the arrest of six of the directors of the company.

The property is now known as *The Elms*, and is being used to house psychologically challenged (I think I have the correct term) male offenders, prior to them being sent on remedial holidays. In fact, it sounds rather like the *Blue House!*

MEMORABLE OTHERS

Bond had a commitment to his fellow agents, but most of all to Queen and Country. There were those alongside him who were heroes, such as other 00s who were killed along the way. There were also villains, often 'taken out' by Bond as part of his work. However, there were other memorable characters who enriched the books and the films. Sometimes they were women, such as Pussy Galore, Honey Ryder, Tatiana Romanova - and so many more. But there was also 'M' and 'Q' and Sheriff J. W. Pepper. They may not have been heroes or villains, but they were memorable.

Likewise with *my* life, and for most people. Many of my memorable people have been patients. They were idiosyncratic, they had a story to tell, they had foibles, or in some other way were unforgettable. I would like you to meet a few of my memorable friends. Friends - disguised as patients.

Memorable Other One.	**A Creature of Habit.**
Memorable Other(s) Two.	**A Mouth Like Two Windows**
Memorable Other Three.	**The Snow Queen**
Memorable Other Four.	**One Dead Cat**
Memorable Other Five.	**Teeth in the Shrubbery**

Memorable Other One.

A Creature of Habit!

Is there *any* country where James Bond has not had adventures? Certain countries immediately bring to mind 007 books and films - Russia, India, New Orleans and the Caribbean, Egypt and Macau are just a few. Wendy and I, too, are privileged to have visited many countries. We have sailed the seven seas, walked on five continents, and been to the Arctic and the Antarctic (which are *not* countries, of course). Having said that, my favourite place, apart from home, is Dovedale in central England. I love the hills, rivers, valleys and peace. I have been walking there twenty-four times now, usually on short breaks. But I do go to many other places. I suppose Wendy and I are adventurers – but we are also creatures of habit. Which brings me to Sid.

* * *

Sid was a committed man. Once he had made up his mind, Sid committed. Absolutely. Completely. And forever.

Sid was committed to Elsie. They had courted in their teens, and had fallen in love. From that moment on, Sid had never looked at another woman, and Elsie had never looked at another man. And when Sid said, "I do," it was not for life, but forever.

Sid was committed to the National Health Service. He worked as a porter in a local hospital, and that too was for life. During the difficult years of the NHS when there were cutbacks and wage freezes and below-inflation pay rises, Sid never considered changing his job. The hospital needed him, and more importantly, the people needed him. Sid was committed to the NHS, and the patients, forever.

At my country practice in rural Norfolk, I saw most of my patients, including Sid, under the NHS. I had to work fairly quickly, because it was 'piece work' and the fee-per-item was not too generous, but I was relatively young and could manage it. As the years passed and I grew older, it was more difficult to keep up the pace - but I too felt a commitment to the NHS, which is a wonderful institution. And then the Government (which was *not* Labour), implemented a 19% pay cut for NHS dentists. 19%! With such a cut in income for the practice, we would have to either stop seeing patients under that system, or reduce the standard of treatment we were delivering.

My solution was for me to stop seeing 'fee paying' patients under the NHS, but to continue with children and those who were on Governments benefits for income reasons. My private fees were lower than those of most dentists in the area, so that those used to paying NHS fees would not find them 'out of reach'. And for those who wanted to stay under the NHS, my young associate dentist would look after them.

Sid? He explained to me that he understood my situation with regard to the fee cut, and he was in a position to pay my fees, and that he liked me as a person and was grateful for the treatment he had received. But he was committed to the NHS. I was not to read anything personal into his decision, but he was totally committed to the NHS. So he would not be coming in to see me again, but would see my associate.

However, Sid continued to be my friend. I expect that he was committed. Walking through the town, I would see him cycling towards me on his bicycle. His eye would fall in my direction and he would smile, brake, and come over to me. "How are you keeping then, Mr. Lawrence?" he would enquire. I was well, thank you, and he told me he was too. "Nothing personal about me not seeing you these days, but I believe in the NHS you see," he explained. I assured him there was no problem at all, and we would proceed to discuss the weather, Norwich City Football Club, and the new housing developments in the town.

Sid was committed to the Labour Party. There were times when the Labour Party was popular and 'riding on the crest of a wave'. And so it should be too, thought Sid. It was Labour who looked after people - not just Sid himself, but the under-privileged, the needy, and the National Health Service.

There were times when the Labour Party was very much out of fashion, but Sid was committed to it. Double digit inflation, high taxation, unions calling their members out on strike - but Sid was committed. Labour. Forever Labour. Whatever. Committed.

Sid was committed to Eastbourne.

"Having a holiday this year, Sid?" I enquired one day.

"Certainly am," he replied, brightening up at the thought. "I take the missus to Eastbourne each year."

"Eastbourne? Every year? Why Eastbourne?' I asked.

"Eastbourne? You can't beat Eastbourne. Best place there is for holidays."

"But why Eastbourne?" I enquired again.

Sid looked at me as though I was stupid. Did I not know that Eastbourne was the best place - in fact, the only really suitable place - for a holiday in England?

"I've been going to Eastbourne for..." Sid was thinking hard now, "for probably about thirty years. I don't know why everybody doesn't go to Eastbourne. Best place in the world. Nowhere to touch it, there ain't."

Sid closed his eyes, and was clearly reliving holiday experiences from 'the best place on earth'.

"There's seven miles of prom that you can walk along. Not that me and me missus walk all of it in one go, or all of it each year. But there it is - seven miles. You can just keep walking, and there's the sea all the way along. Wonderful. And then there's Mrs. Scroggin's Bed and Breakfast. Always go to Mrs.

Scroggins, we do. Lovely place, and the best full English breakfast you can get anywhere. I don't know why everybody doesn't go and stay with Mrs. Scroggins. Eastbourne - *the* most wonderful place."

Clearly, Sid was totally captivated with the charms of Eastbourne, and had been for many years. But did he know what the rest of the world had to offer - Mediterranean sunshine, the golden beaches of the Caribbean, the chateaux of the Loire Valley.....

"Sid, have you *always* gone to Eastbourne? Have you never ever tried *anywhere* else?" I had to ask.

"Well, yes, we did. It was a long time ago now, when we were younger, and we thought we ought to try somewhere else. Just to see, you know. So we went to Bournemouth for a week."

"And how was Bournemouth?" I enquired.

"Bournemouth? Bournemouth wasn't no good at all," said Sid sadly. "It rained in Bournemouth. So the next year we went back to Eastbourne. Lovely place Eastbourne. Always go there. Nowhere like it. I don't know why everybody doesn't go to Eastbourne."

Memorable Other(s) Two.

A Mouth Like Two Windows

Auric Goldfinger was a one man success story. Some people are like that - everything they touch turns to gold. King Midas was such a man. Literally.

Some of my patients seemed to have that touch too. I used to be a trifle envious of them but, as time went on, I changed my mind. Being short of money can cause anxiety, but having lots of money does not bring happiness. Quality of life can be experienced by people with little money, and deep unhappiness by those with a fortune. Read the newspapers! But I have known really happy people who have very little. I have also known those who have been very successful in business. Decent people like Jane and Chris.

* * *

"Expensive? No way. Your mouth is like two windows!"

* * *

Jane and her husband Chris were new patients to the practice, but we instantly became friends. Well, not the sort of friends who spent time together socialising, but we enjoyed each other's company, mainly in the surgery.

They were local people, as far as I can recall. Living about ten miles from the surgery on the outskirts of a small town on the north Norfolk coast, they drove almost past the surgery each day in order to arrive at the industrial estate where they worked, in a village on the other side of town. But they had never called in to see me before.

There are two major reasons why people stay away from the dentist. Firstly, many people are just too busy, and so long as there is no pain, their teeth can wait. This was Jane. She and Chris were busy. So busy. But now she had pain, and realised that several of her teeth really needed attention.

The second reason for many people avoiding the dentist, is that they are scared. Some people would say 'petrified'. This too was Jane. The very thought of a needle penetrating her gums would cause a massive flow of adrenalin and she would go pale and feel unable to move. And that was just the thought.

But there comes a point when the pain is so bad that even the most fearful person will make an appointment. At such times, personal support is more than helpful, and Chris had said that he would come along with her.

Jane was pale, nervously looking round, and sat down in the dental chair slowly and reluctantly. Chris was relaxed, smiling and supportive. For some reason I had placed a huge cane peacock chair in the corner of my surgery, and Chris sat there like the Shah of Persia, speaking encouraging and comforting words to Jane.

"You're doing fine dear. What a lovely bright surgery. Close your eyes and imagine you're on a sunny beach."

It was my usual practice to sit on a chair some distance from the patient so that they would not feel threatened, and ask them to tell me anything that was wrong, and what they might like me to do about it. I placed a chair just to the left of Chris, smiled at him and then Jane, and asked what I could do for them.

"I'm in pain. Just get on with it," said Jane.

"Have a look round," said Chris, "Stop the pain as soon as possible, and then tell us *all* that needs doing, and we'll come back. And she would like to be knocked out - get everything done in one go if possible. We're very busy people, but we will take time to get Jane's teeth put right now that we've come."

So I charted everything that was there, and everything that was not there. Antibiotics and painkillers would alleviate the discomfort that had brought them in, given a little time. But a root filling was required to save the tooth, and several crowns and bridges, in addition to fillings, would be needed if they really wanted to get her dentition into good shape. And she would need an intravenous sedation so that she was unaware of the treatment at the time.

"How much?" said Chris. "No need for a breakdown by items or any explanation. I think I can really trust you, so give me a figure and tell me how many appointments."

"OK," I replied. "The information you have asked for is £4,250 and four appointments. I can appreciate that you don't want to spend too long sitting and listening to a lengthy explanation and breakdown of costs, but the treatment will involve several crowns, two bridges, a root treatment and a few fillings. I'm sure you have some questions."

"None at all. I like you and I trust you," said Chris. "When can you get Jane in?"

"*How* much!" said Jane. It was more of an exclamation than a question. "That seems awfully expensive."

"Expensive? No way. Your mouth is like two windows," said Chris.

"Your wife's mouth is like two windows? That sounds more like a mother-in-law joke. I can't see the connection," I replied.

So Chris explained. The two of them had started out in business together making small double-glazed windows. They became quite busy, and so took on another person to help them. Then they became busier still, and employed several more staff and widened their range of products. Soon after, they had to extend the premises and take on further staff. There were about one hundred now, and they were working flat out.

"Thank goodness for Asia," said Chris, and seeing that I looked completely non-plussed by this, continued. "We seem to be having small groups of Asian gentlemen visiting the factory almost every day. They come up from London because we're so much cheaper. Norfolk, you see. And they come on behalf of councils and order double-glazed units by the hundred. Thank goodness for Asia. They soon paid for my Jag, but I have precious little time to enjoy it. And by the way, Jane's mouth will cost us about two windows. Your bill is what we get for two decent windows. No problem at all."

Then he grinned broadly.

"Put your money where your mouth is," he exclaimed with a roar of laughter. "Get it? - or should I say, 'Put your money where *your wife's* mouth is?' That's what I say."

That was way back in the 1980s, but a memorable time, and within a couple of months, Jane's dentition was restored, they sold at least two windows, paid on the way out and made a six-monthly appointment for an examination. And then Chris booked himself in, and had a little under a 'window' of treatment.

They were great 'people people.' Some of their staff came in as patients, and clearly regarded Chris and Jane as genuine friends, as well as respecting them as their employers. Each time any of the office staff had a birthday, Jane took the whole office out to lunch to celebrate. And Christmas was a riot!

I felt sorry that Chris and Jane had to work such long hours, and that they were not able to enjoy the Jaguar car or have reasonable leisure time. This seemed to be a common occurrence amongst patients who were in business. In the early days they would put all their time and energy into their work in order to drive it along and give it some momentum. Then, when they wanted to slow down and enjoy the income, they could not do so because the business was driving them along. I saw a number of such people have breakdowns, and head off to the Mediterranean on doctor's orders. And dentists were not immune from this, which was why I always spent most of each weekend with my family, took them away on holiday during the summer, and quite often took my wife out to lunch on a weekday. And when I was forty, I went onto a four-day week. I liked my work, loved my patients, but prioritised my family and my leisure.

However, things looked up for Chris and Jane, as they became friendly with a bookie and his wife. A bookie, if you are unfamiliar with the term, is a turf accountant. A turf accountant, if you are unfamiliar with the term, is a gentleman who takes bets, usually on horse races though these days on many other sports, election results, weather - almost anything where the element of chance is involved. This opened up life in a much fuller way for Chris and Jane, and they would speak of visits to European cities and beach holidays in the sun with their new friends.

"Could you take on our friends, Jeff and Linda?" asked Chris as he was leaving the surgery one day. Of course I could. Within the week, both had booked in, though separately.

Jeff duly attended for his first appointment, and I was quite taken aback at his appearance. His jeans looked as though he had been gardening, then changed the oil in the car - and spilt some. His shirt matched! On top, was a well-worn jacket. He marched over to me with a broad smile and an extended hand. We shook, and I knew that I would enjoy conversation with Jeff.

"I must apologise for my state of attire," he said with a grin, and went on to explain. "I come into town here for the auctions at the market on Mondays, and it seemed best to arrange to see you at the same time. The auctions - best to appear poor there. Not just for the auction itself, but for informal trading at some of the stalls. Hence the outfit. Always seems to work."

I took X-rays and examined his teeth. He needed to come back for a few visits and his treatment would cost a few hundred pounds.

"I'll pay the lot now, if that's OK," he said, and proceeded to reach inside his jacket. Right breast pocket - the thickest bundle of fifty pound notes I had ever seen. He counted off the appropriate number, and after replacing the remainder, extracted an equally thick wad of twenty pound notes from the left hand pocket. After replacing those left (most), a thick pile of tenners was drawn out of his jeans, right side, and one of these concluded the settlement. "No need for the fivers," said Jeff.

I would normally have expected the patient to pay at reception, but a number of businessmen who dealt largely in cash, mainly very used banknotes, seemed to think I would prefer them pushed straight into my hand in the surgery. Can't think why!

A week or so later Linda presented for her appointment. She was exquisitely dressed, with make-up perfectly applied, and spoke like the lady on the BBC news channel. She needed little treatment, and asked for her account to be sent to her husband.

* * *

I must have mentioned my Christian faith to Chris at some point, though I cannot recall when. But it obviously made some sort of impact, as he came back to me about it, and in a curious way.

When my first marriage broke down, a family in the town where I was later to have a practice invited me to stay with them, while I tried to bring the marriage and family together again. Unsuccessfully. I was with them for six months, and will be eternally grateful to them for the love, care and support they provided. I also went to their church on Sundays.

I struggled rather in that church. Pews, all stand up for a hymn, all sit down for a prayer, one man with a dog collar doing all the stuff at the front was neither my conviction nor my choice. (Having said that, they had a new minister some years later, and everything livened up.) When I moved into the little rose-coloured cottage in the country later that year, I continued going to their church, until... It was a weekday and for some reason I felt I should go and have a look at a Wesleyan chapel in the town. It was open and I walked in. What a strange experience - it was as if a divine arm reached down, embraced me, and told me I had just entered my new home. The following Sunday I went to one of their services, and I stayed there for twenty-five years.

There were around thirty of us meeting there. There was no 'minister', but three or four of us either led the meeting or preached, and others prayed, read scriptures or whatever they felt was right. It was a small town of around four and a half thousand in population, and there were seven churches. And then the Wesleyan started to grow. One year, fifty-two new people confessed conversion to Christ, and joined us from unchurched backgrounds. Our chapel could no longer accommodate us, and so we rented the town hall. We grew further in numbers, and next rented a 'drill hall'.

One Sunday morning I had parked our car and was walking to the drill hall. I waited for a car to pass before crossing the road, but it stopped. It was a Jaguar. The driver's window was lowered, and Chris smiled up at me.

"Are you off to church? Is that a Bible you're holding?"

Yes, I was, and yes, it was.

"I want to talk to you about your religion," said Chris. "Is that the right word? Or is it your faith? Anyway, I know from what you've said that you have this faith, and it's very real to you, isn't it? It shows, you see. So I want us to talk, because I want to know if it's real. Now don't misunderstand me, cos I don't want to join your church. I don't think I do, and I don't think I will. But I want to know - is it true, or is it not? I think I need to know."

I think a lot of people need to know, and are in that position. Chris was very honest. He did not really believe the Christian faith - but he was curious, and thought he might be wrong. So having found someone who was convinced of their faith, he decided to try and find out for himself. I suggested we meet up sometime for a drink, or a curry, but he said he was busy for a while.

Our church continued growing as people from the town and surrounding villages were converted to Christ, joined us and threw themselves into the work of the fellowship. We now numbered nearly three hundred and were renting the High School, when an old bus station came up for sale. The church had two thousand pounds in the bank, and the asking price was one hundred and seventy-five thousand pounds. We bid the asking price, our offer was accepted, and we started praying like we never had before, for a target of four hundred and thirty-five thousand to include refurbishing it. To cut a long story short, the money came in, the building was totally renovated and refurbished, and in 1992 the work was completed. We praised God, celebrated in style, and had a dinner one evening to which we invited friends from outside the church.

I hadn't seen Chris and Jane for a while, but noticed they were coming in for examinations the following week. I invited them to the dinner, and they joined my wife and I for the evening. Chris was interested in what the church was doing by way of projects to help people, but we were unable to find a time to meet up to discuss the more important issues. As we left, Jane took me to one side and with lowered voice, enquired whether she could ask a question about the church. Of course she could.

"Where do you bury your dead?" she asked in a hushed voice. She had noticed that the converted bus station did not have a graveyard. In fact, the town graveyard was immediately adjacent to our new church building. I lowered my voice to match hers, and said,

"Shhh. We throw them over the hedge." She looked horrified, and then realised I was joking and grinned.

"Seriously, we have a funeral service like any other church, usually celebrating the person's life, and then go to the crematorium or town graveyard." We walked to our cars, said that we should meet up again as a foursome for dinner, and bade each other goodnight.

That was the last time I saw Chris and Jane together. In fact, I did not see either of them for a long time. Some of their staff continued to come to the surgery, and one of them told me that they were no longer living together. I heard later that the business was in Jane's name, and that when Chris arrived for work one morning, his Jaguar was taken from him by one of the staff, and Jane told him he was sacked. Mobile phones were the size of small bricks in those days, and Chris' phone, like his Jaguar, was company property and was taken back. He had to walk to our town, and find a taxi to get home.

A few years later, Jane came back to the surgery, the first of a number of visits. She sometimes arrived in her Porsche with a personalised registration, and sometimes in her BMW with a personalised registration. She spoke of her new home, of how she was enjoying single life again, and of the joys of having an orangery. But she seemed strangely incomplete without Chris.

Chris and Jane (not your real names, of course, but you will recognize yourselves) - I enjoyed your visits, your warmth of personality, humour and conversation. You were patients from heaven. You enriched my life. I wish you well.

Memorable Other Three.

The Snow Queen

The Countess Lisl von Schlaf, played by Cassandra Harris in *For Your Eyes Only (1981)*, is a sophisticated, aristocratic lady, attired in an expensive evening gown. It is one of those late bedroom scenes, when she suddenly exclaims, "Me nightie's slipping." It was an interesting moment, and Bond comes out with a memorable one-liner. I sometimes thought of the Countess when visited by a lady whose culture was all part of *the races*.

* * *

The Snow Queen arrived for her appointment dressed, as usual, in an ankle-length satin evening gown. She swept into the surgery accompanied by her smartly dressed husband, to whom she passed her stole and small sequined evening bag. It was 11 a.m.

At her first appointment with me, Mrs. Shirley Jones had explained that she and her husband were 'racing people'. Newmarket, Great Yarmouth, Fakenham - they were always there, and dressed appropriately. One might have thought that she resided in Great Walsingham Hall, or at least, Lesser Barningham Manor or similar, but her records indicated Walnut Cottage, The Lane, Bogswood. I was sure that Bogswood was a very pleasant place to live.

Softly spoken, but with the air of sophistication that can accompany the idle rich, Mrs. Jones confided in me concerning her underlying problem. "I am so frightfully apprehensive of you people," she whispered. "I really need a general anaesthetic. I don't suppose that could be arranged?"

I explained that, although I had once administered literally hundreds of general anaesthetics, members of the dental profession were no longer legally permitted to do so.

"How dreadful," said the Snow Queen. "How frightfully boorish of them."

I agreed with her, but proceeded to explain that I was qualified to administer an intravenous (needle-in-the-arm) sedative, that would not only induce a sense of well-being approaching mild euphoria, but also cause significant amnesia. She might even forget that she had been to the dentist.

"Admirable. So pleased. The cost will be no problem. I shall arrange to see you as soon as possible." And after I had checked her medical history and been through the pre- and post-op instructions, she floated out of the surgery.

* * *

The Snow Queen? It was the dress. Or dresses. They were always of ankle length, and invariably in white or cream. And elegant. My staff were unanimous - she was 'The Snow Queen'.

"It's the races," she explained again. "We are racing people, and one really has to dress for the occasion, you see. And for so many other occasions too."

* * *

"I have simply starved myself," said the Snow Queen, gazing up from the chair with a pained look. "I'm famished. Dreadfully. But it just has to be," she almost purred with her velvety tones.

The chair was tilted back, and a tourniquet applied to her left arm. I gently inserted the syringe into a prominent vein in her anterior cubital fossa, the slightly depressed vein-rich area near the elbow, and favoured for such procedures. I eased the midazolam into her blood stream.

The Snow Queen's pupils slowly dilated, and rolled upwards a degree. At the same time her eyelids descended to cover half the eye itself. At this point, I liked to reassure the patient that all was well, and so I gently enquired, "How are you feeling, Mrs. Jones?"

Her response took us all by surprise, and remained one of those closely guarded matters of confidentiality.

"Actually darlin', Oi'm feelin' quoite pissed," said our local lovely. "Quoite pissed," repeated Shirley, our very Norfolk member of the racing set. Very Norfolk.

In fact, she sounded frightfully inebriated. Frightfully so.

Memorable Other Four.

One Dead Cat

For a Bond aficionado, there are lots of little quirks with the film characters. For instance, there are eight actors who have appeared in Bond movies more than once - and playing a different character in each. A particularly interesting example is Charles Gray. He appeared in 1967 in *You Only Live Twice,* as Australian intelligence officer Richard 'Dikko' Henderson, an ally of Bond's. But in *Diamonds Are Forever (1971),* he plays Blofeld, Bond's arch-enemy.

In the opening scene of the latter film, Blofeld is using surgery to produce look-alikes. Bond crashes in, and mistakenly kills the wrong man, a look-alike. Later in the story, Bond scales a high-rise building where Blofeld is based - and again mistakenly kills a look-alike. Of course, Bond eventually gets the right man, as you would expect. I wonder if the prison officer, Jack Flint, had ever seen this film?

* * *

"I might be a prison officer, but I sat down at the table and wept buckets. Just couldn't stop," said Jack.

* * *

Jack and Julie Flint used to live near me, though I did not know them at the time. My first marriage had hit crisis and I had rented a property just out of the city. Jack and Julie had lived down the road from me.

Those had been difficult days indeed, as many readers will understand. And worse was to come, and again, many of you will be able to identify with me in that. But as I have already written, I was tremendously blessed, helped, and encouraged by a lovely couple who invited me to become part of their family for as long as I wanted. And so I left the village where Jack and Julie lived, without ever meeting them.

After living with the family for six months, and realising that my marriage was not going to come together again, I bought a small cottage just two miles from the property I had rented, and started making a new life for myself. They were sad days, but I felt there really was light at the end of the tunnel, even if I could not yet see it. I was determined not to be swallowed up by the darkness.

Just how does one survive such times, and come through with a smile on one's face and into a future that's even better. I will digress slightly here from the story of Jack and Julie, and briefly say how I handled the situation. Firstly, and predictably for me, I tried to deepen my relationship with the God we read about in the Bible, and who had changed my whole life many years previously. I made sure that I put time aside each day just to spend with him - reading the Bible, meditating on what I had read, and praying. Praying? - praise, worship, thanking him, and making a few requests for other people and sometimes for myself. Secondly, I launched out into activities that would occupy my mind and my energy, and be fulfilling as well as giving a sense of achievement. I chose colour schemes for the different rooms in the little cottage I had bought, and set about applying them. I also recalled the joy of collecting eggs from my parents' hens when I was a young boy, and bought chickens and started collecting eggs again. Thirdly, I tried to maintain old friendships as well as developing new ones. I learnt to cook and found that dinner parties were a fun way of deepening relationships, as well as finding the creative act of cooking therapeutic in itself.

Just over a year later, I started a branch practice in the small market town where my host family lived. I worked there on a very part-time basis at first, going in for a half-day every day, but in less than a year, had a full-time associate dentist working there with me. And after four years or so, I sold my city practice and worked solely in the little town out in the county.

One day, Jack and Julie came to my new practice, which was only five miles further from Norwich than they were. They pointed out to me that it was so much quicker and easier to get to me than going into the city itself. Jack and I found we had a common interest, or perhaps by this time, history, in having played squash at the same club many years previously. We had not known each other then, but had a mutual friend who had also been a member of the club, and who had such an amazing personality that we were continually remembering anecdotes concerning him. "Do you remember him doing a bungee jump off that crane in the centre of the city?" and "Did you hear about him going round pubs doing fifty press-ups on one hand?" and "Do you remember how he had the words 'John F. Howard, Builder and Squash Coach' written along the side of his truck?"

Jack worked as a prison officer, and I realised that I had not knowingly met many such people before. In fact, I had met just two, and they were each memorable, though for completely different reasons. The first was simply a *prospective* prison officer, and was at school with me. We were known by our surnames only there, followed by initials, so I was either 'Lawrence' or 'Lawrence B R' not only to the masters, but also to my friends. I was never really friendly with 'Waller M S', but we were in the same year, and so there was a certain bond. From his early teens, Waller had just one ambition - to be a prison officer.

Now, there might be nothing remarkable in wanting to spend ones life looking after prisoners, except that Waller's best friend was 'Milton B. M.'. They lived near each other in the same Norfolk seaside town, and may even have been close buddies before coming to the grammar school. Milton however, was, as a youngster, naughty, and as a teenager, a young villain. I thought he was probably a psychopath. In the second form, he at one time occupied the desk in front of mine, and, when the master was not looking, would lob a comic over his shoulder onto my desk. He would then give a loud cough that sounded remarkably like the word, 'Lawrence', leaving me to quickly hide it in my desk, fearful that it would be seen, and that *I* would get into trouble. Which was Milton's intention, of course. But by the third form he was in serious trouble for taking protection money from first-formers who did not want to be beaten up, and whilst in the fourth form, was arrested by the police for a break-in at a tobacconist's, where several thousand cigarettes were stolen. He, and another teenager who did not attend our school, were found guilty. Milton was expelled from the school.

The last time I heard news of Milton was when I was in my fourth year of training at the London Hospital in Whitechapel. By this time Waller was working as a prison officer. I had settled into a leather armchair in the athenaeum (men's common room), and gathered a few newspapers to try and catch up on recent news. And there in the Daily Express, was the story of a Norfolk man, Barry Milton. Yes - his first name was Barry. He and another man had driven down to Brighton and raided a jeweler's shop. Leaving the town in their minivan, they were chased by a police patrol car. Milton was defiantly firing at them with a shotgun through the minivan window, as they careered off the road and crashed. He was arrested while staggering across a field of potatoes, still clutching the shotgun. I looked for some follow-up to this in the national press, but was unable to find anything. However, it certainly looked as though he would be receiving a lengthy custodial sentence, and the questions that kept entering my mind were - would Milton meet up again with his old chum Waller? If so, what sort of relationship would there be between these two men? Maybe one of them will read this book; if so, please get in touch, as I've so many questions.

The other prison officer that I had met was Ernest Garfield Wareham, who told me he was a 'discipline officer' at the Guys Marsh Borstal just outside Shaftesbury, the Dorset town where I worked for five years. The boys used to come into the practice where I worked, and make remarks such as 'nice pad here' as they entered the surgery. That was one place I saw them. The other place was when I was driving south from Shaftesbury towards Sturminster Newton, when we would pass the institution on our left. It was not unusual to observe some of the inmates sitting in the ditch by the roadside, smoking cigarettes and chatting up the local girls. Mr. Wareham was a man of few words, and when I asked him how long he had been in the prison service, paused before telling me that it was four years.

"What did you do before that?" I enquired.

Again there was a thoughtful pause before he disclosed, "I was a professional wrestler." And that, perhaps, accounted for the absence of his upper front teeth.

"Were you ever on television?" I asked.

"Most Saturday afternoons, but not all. Had to have some recovery times in that game," he volunteered without so much as a smile.

"I expect the boys are quite impressed with that," I remarked. "But I always used to watch wrestling with my parents on the Saturday Grandstand programme on television, until I went to London. I don't remember an Ernest Wareham. Did you use another name?"

Once more there was a pause, and this time longer than the previous two. Then,

"I was *The Slasher*! And don't you dare tell the boys, cos I'd never hear the end of it."

* * *

Jack was a well-built, athletic tough guy. His wife was a lady who dressed elegantly and spoke without the local accent. But Jack was tough. There would be no nonsense from the inmates when Jack was around. And so the following story he related stayed with me, and even as I write, I can hear him telling it to me.

Jack and Julie had a cat. It was not a remarkable cat aesthetically - a tabby, but truly 'one of the family', and had been with them for several years. And then the cat went missing. At first they assumed it was up to some business away from home, as cats do. After two days they searched for it and called it, but to no avail.

That evening they were having friends round to dinner, and Julie spent much of the day preparing. Jack was off duty, and whilst busying himself around the house, was interrupted by a ring at the doorbell. Answering the door, Jack found himself staring at a neighbour who was himself staring at Jack with a deadpan expression. Then he looked down and muttered, "Is your cat alright Jack?"

Jack explained that the cat had been missing for a couple of days, and immediately began to sense what his neighbour had come to tell him.

"It's been beside the road for a day or two," he said. "Tabby. I couldn't believe it was yours, but thought I ought to come and enquire."

Almost overcome with sadness, Jack walked with his neighbour to where the remains of the cat lay beside the road. Jack lovingly carried the rather tatty carcase of the cat back to his home, and told Julie, who became very pale and quiet. They buried the cat in their back garden, and went back indoors. Jack went to their bedroom, sat down and wept.

That evening, their dinner guests duly arrived, and they served pre-dinner drinks, though the death of the cat totally preoccupied them, especially Jack. They sat at the table, and Julie brought in their starters, but at this point, Jack could contain himself no longer.

"I might be a prison officer, but I sat at the table and wept buckets. Just couldn't stop," said Jack. "So I left the room, went upstairs, and broke down. Julie explained to our guests."

He proceeded to tell me he wept and wept for a further two days. Julie told him he really needed to get a grip on his life again, and they were sitting down together, having a real heart to heart, when...

There was a click from the kitchen, followed by the unmistakable sound of the cat flap swinging. And there was Tabby, significantly skinnier than before and clearly asking to be fed!

* * *

After telling me the story, Jack paused and said, "I wonder whose cat I buried!"

Memorable Other Five.

Teeth in the Shrubbery!

Colonel Rosa Klebb was a leading agent of *SPECTRE*. She was mean, unsmiling, and had lethal, poisonous, spiky shoes. But not every female villain was in the style of Rosa Klebb. Hench-woman May Day, played by Grace Jones wearing a short black leather tunic and thigh boots, in *A View To A Kill (1985)*, was worth a second look. Likewise Xenia Onatopp, played by Famke Janssen, in *Goldeneye (1995)*, caused many a chap to pause the video and hit 'Replay'. The most beautiful Russian agent in the Bond films, in my opinion, was Barbara Bach play-ing Anya Amasova in *The Spy Who Loved Me (1977)*. I think that Ringo Starr would agree with me, because he married the lady.

More locally, I was informed that there was a female arch-villain called Mrs. Grimble. But after hearing the whole story, I am not so sure it was not Mrs. Gumm.

* * *

"She threw my teeth out of the window - and they landed in the shrubbery," said Mrs. Winifred Gumm of Aegel House, fight-ing back the tears. "The staff spent ages looking for them."

* * *

With the arrival of a new patient, there are certain scenarios that immediately cause warning lights to flash. One such is the patient who embarks on, "And then I went to Mr. Smith, and he carried out such and such treatment, and that didn't work. And then I went to Mr. Jones and he did such and such, and *that* didn't work. And then I went to Mrs. Williams...." Another is the patient who, having entered the surgery, starts unwrapping a package, and then forlornly holds up a bag containing several sets of false teeth. Each set has been provided by a previous dentist. The teeth didn't fit. They hurt. They were too big. They were too small. Too light. Too dark. And having been to a succession of dentists, yours truly is now the next in line.

Mrs. Winifred Gumm - she had been to 'Mr. Smith' and 'Mr. Jones' and 'Mrs. Williams' and more. The result? A large polythene bag containing innumerable sets of false teeth. I was doomed!

"You see," she explained, "Mrs. Williams in Frippingham tried to make them smaller, but then they didn't show and people thought I wasn't wearing any. I went to Mrs. Williams because, before that, I had been to Mr. Jones in Falthorpe, and he had made them too big. The other people I live with laughed at me, and said I looked like a horse. I felt so silly. I went to Mr. Jones because before that I had been to Mr. Smith in Norwich, and he had made them with wings on. They stuck in and hurt. I went to Mr. Smith because Mr. Worth in Waltworth, who I went to before that, had made teeth that moved around......."

I politely inspected the bag of teeth.

"I'm not sure that I can do any better," I offered. "You obviously have a very difficult mouth, and I'm not sure I can improve on what the others have done."

But Mrs. Gumm had heard that I was a born-again Christian, and she now produced her trump card.

"But I've *prayed* about it, Mr. Lawrence, and I really believe that you are the person who can help me."

Now that is a difficult one to answer!

So I reluctantly agreed to 'do my best' and 'under the NHS' as that would cost her nothing, as she was not exactly wealthy, and would also mean that I would not have to 'give Mrs.

Gumm her money back' if she was dissatisfied. She positively beamed at me.

One month and four appointments later, Mrs. Gumm walked out of my surgery, smiling at the world with her new dentures.

"I knew you would make me good teeth," she gushed. "You see - I *prayed* about it."

Two days later she was back in my chair. "Just a tiny bit off here where it's rubbing."

Two more days later she was back again. "A weeny bit off here please."

The following week she returned. "A minute bit off here please."

Two days later. "A little sore at the back."

Two days later. "A little sore at the front."

The following week. "They don't feel quite right."

Two days later. "There're still not quite right."

Two days later. "Almost there."

The following week. "Just a tiny bit off here where it's rubbing."

Two days later. "A weeny bit off here please."

And then she stopped for a week or so.

"There's a lady to see you about Mrs. Gumm," said Maureen on reception. I had a few minutes and suggested she came through to the surgery.

"I work at Aegel House," said the lady. "As a care assistant there. They said I ought to come and explain what's happened."

Aegel House, the residential home for the elderly, was just a short walk down the road from the surgery. For a few years I had thought it was *Angel* House, and had written that on several of the residents notes when they came for treatment. No - it was Aegel. Who was Aegel, I wondered? Only recently have I discovered that Aegel was a Saxon farmer whose homestead was known as Aegel's Ham, and later as Aylsham. It is recorded in the Domesday Book, where the population was similar to that of a couple of decades ago. But since then, houses have been built by the hundreds. After the Norman Conquest, Aylsham became Crown property, until Charles I pawned it to the Corporation of the City of London. He was never able to redeem it. Eventually, it was passed on in its entirety to the Earls of Buckinghamshire, who already owned the nearby hamlet of Blickling. And then it was transferred to the National Trust, who are its guardians today. Blickling Hall, a stately home, was once the residence of the Boleyn family, and the Buckinghamshire Arms stands a stone's throw away and assuages the thirsts and satisfies the appetites of many of the Hall's visitors each year.

Now back to Mrs. Gumm, who was not in good health. It was not just that she hobbled with a stick, but "She gets fixations, she does," said Karen, the carer. "It's been one thing after another, and she goes on and on, she does. Everyone got really fed up with it, but the thing she has had about her teeth for the last six months has been too much for some of the other residents. Moan, moan, moan all day long." Karen paused, and let out a long sigh.

"Anyway, she gets back from your surgery after each of her visits, and takes her teeth out and puts them on the arm of her chair in the resident's lounge. 'Put 'em back in', some of the others shout out. And one of them, Mrs. Grimble, threatened to 'do something serious' if she didn't put them back in, or leave them in her own room. And Mrs. Grimble has been really upset recently, and...."

We were interrupted by Maureen entering the surgery.

"Mrs. Gumm has just walked in and asked to see you," said Maureen, at which Karen the carer said she had better leave, and stepped briskly out through the surgery door.

"I'll show her in," said Maureen.

Enter Mrs. Gumm, who was clearly upset.

"She threw my teeth out of the window - and they landed in the shrubbery," said Mrs. Winifred Gumm, fighting back the tears. The staff spent ages looking for them."

She thought they had been damaged. Would I make some new ones? She was sure I would make some that would be absolutely perfect, because the last set had been 'almost'. But I declined. I was tempted to say that I had *prayed* about it, but resisted. There was another dentist in the town, and I had heard that he was good. Yes, really good. Especially at false teeth. Made them perfect, he did.

So Mrs. Gumm bade me farewell, and set off for the dentist who made false teeth that were perfect. Usually. Maybe. Perhaps.

And some time later, Mavis, another of the staff from Aegel House attended for treatment, and related how Mrs. Gumm had moaned and groaned about her teeth, and how much they hurt, and how many times she had been back to see me. Day after day she would sit with her teeth balanced on the arm of her chair, grinning toothlessly at the other residents as she wittered on and on about her dental troubles. Mrs. Grimble had told her to shut up a hundred times, until the day that she could stand it no more.

Waiting until Mrs. Gumm appeared asleep, and hobbling along with her walking stick, she snatched up the teeth and made for the door. There was a shout from Mrs. Gumm, who picked up her stick and struggled out of her chair.

"Give me m' teef," she shouted as best she could. "I want m' teef back."

Mrs. Grimble was well ahead and passed through the door and into the corridor, but with Mrs. Gumm in (fairly) hot pursuit.

"I want m' teef. Give 'em back," shouted Mrs. Gumm, nearly in tears.

"But Mrs. Grimble was opening a window in the corridor," said Mavis. "Next thing, we saw her throw the teeth as far as she could, even though she's got arthritis. 'Good riddance' she shouted, and hobbled back to her room. Mrs. Gumm was in tears, and Mrs. Rogers, the manager, had us all out looking for the teeth. They had been thrown from the upstairs, you see. It was a few days before they turned up, and we think that the person who found them actually hid them quick, because we were *all* fed up with it. Now she's had a new set made by that other dentist, and she's moaning and going back there almost every day. But," said Mavis, with an impish grin, "She hasn't left them on the arm of the chair any more, and Mrs. Grimble sits opposite her and watches her like a hawk!"

Team Barrie

As a young man, I would occasionally visit the cinema. At the close of the film, the cast would scroll from the bottom of the screen, starting with the stars, and moving on to others such as stuntmen, designers, and other people who played a vital role in the production. However, I recently took two of my granddaughters to watch a popular film, and wondered who some of the actors were. I waited patiently at the conclusion of the film - and waited. I am still not sure who the stars were, as lists of technical people seemed to pass by interminably. However, all those acknowledged in this section are stars. I will try to cover them without being tedious, whilst begging forgiveness of any who have slipped through the memory net somehow.

I have worked with so many dentists, but Sandy Pitt-Steele was *my* dentist during my teenage years, and contributed more than he could ever have realised to my own future in the profession. The clinical staff of the London Hospital Dental Institute were, generally, inspiring, and my fellow students, known as *Blue Year*, were a fabulous crowd.

I qualified and became an associate for five years at the practice of Reg Carnall in Shaftesbury in Dorset. Thank you Reg - you helped me so much as I tried to find my feet in dental practice. And then I moved back to Norfolk, and had a succession of associates. I am so grateful to each of them. I will just mention them by first name, and thereby protect the identities of the (very few) clowns and idiots amongst them. Bob, Andy, Tony, John, Christine, Raymond, Martin, Chris, Mark, Jim, John, Russell and Nita. Thank you, guys, for having been such an integral part of my practices, and contributing to the richness of my life as a dental surgeon.

Dental hygienists became an important part of the dental team at each of my practices from the mid-1970s. Jo, Sharon, Jeanie, Derek and Ged - you were such invaluable members of the team, and the majority of my patients really loved you. Each of you. And I am so grateful to you.

Receptionists are critical to the success, or otherwise, of a dental practice. They give the 'first impression' as they answer the telephone or greet the new arrival entering the waiting room. Miss Elizabeth Cooke at the Shaftesbury practice was to me, as a young associate, the quintessential dental receptionist. However, my own receptionists excelled, combining warmth with professionalism, and at the same time being something of a 'pastor' to the younger members of the team. Daphne was my first receptionist when I opened the single surgery in Norwich, and was still there when I sold the five surgery practice it had grown to be, to my senior associate, Jim Peirson. Daphne was a fantastic 'people person' and was an invaluable asset to this young fang-pranger who was still finding his way in life and practice. Dawn was not only receptionist, but also decorator, plumber, cleaner, manager, pastor, and Jack-of-all-trades at my Aylsham practice. Dawn, you were truly appreciated. Fran was amazing, as she sped and gyrated around the waiting room, and tore along corridors, often shrieking with laughter. She was fun. Maureen was the next to occupy that reception desk, and knew so many local people, which was a great asset. And later there was Hilary, who I still see frequently, as she helps keep Aylsham Tesco running properly, very much as she did *Woodview Dental Health Practice*. Christine Martin is another lady who was enormously appreciated in reception at my Norwich practice, and who we now encounter when attending Cromer hospital for cataract operations and such like. Sarah Crowe was very much in the background whilst nursing, but emerged as a real personality when she moved to reception. And she knew absolutely *everything* there was to know about Liverpool Football Club.

We pioneered in dental hygiene and education. It was new, almost *avant garde*, so we were entering unknown territory to some extent. Dawn was my first dental health educator, and she was brilliant. Likewise Angie, who followed her (and who recently came up to me at the Royal Norfolk Show to say Hello and catch up on news). She too was a great asset to the practice.

Dental nurses were indispensable. Most were fantastic. Some were very unsuited to such work, and did not stay too long. But most quickly became part of the team, and are still appreciated today. I have had so many work for me, in so many surgeries, but I will mention a few who were especially memorable and/or valued. Tish, Belinda, Chris, Jan, Sally, Sue, Pam, Vicky, Jacqueline, Sue, Amanda, Karen, Frank, Louise, Sam, Sandra, Jill, Caroline, Melissa, Julie, Tania... and so many more.

There are team members who are upfront, high profile, and known to all. Equally, there are those who are so much in the background that they are easily overlooked. Laboratory technicians are largely unseen and unheard. Over the years, I came to really appreciate the skills of certain men who constructed gold and porcelain crowns, and dentures that could not be distinguished from natural teeth. Lou Thurston has been mentioned in the first chapter, and was a true craftsman. In Norwich, I appreciated a number of dental technicians more than they probably realised. Adrian Howman, Peter Cook, Peter Newton, Chris Newton, Brian Bulpitt, Dick Butler, Les Gotts, Richard Lyst and Steve Myers are those who were especially appreciated and who I was always pleased to recommend. Other background people were book-keepers (Jack Howard and Barry Halford), cleaners (so many over the years), and dental engineers who would quickly appear when a surgery 'broke down'. Geoffrey Simpson was the star, as well as a good friend.

Where would I have been without patients? Unemployed, or

perhaps, writing books at a much earlier age? At this point, I could write lists going well into three figures, and probably four. Or five. Phillip Clarke, private detective, was typical of so many in that he quickly became a friend. Not that we went to the pub together, or socialised much outside the surgery, but when I saw his name on my day list, I would smile and look forward to seeing him. "Hi Phillip" and "Hi Barrie" were so much more appropriate than, "Good afternoon, Mr. Clarke." And likewise for many others. I am tempted to list those who gave me leaving presents when I retired, or who still send me Christmas cards, but suffice to say I really loved multitudes of people who were *friends disguised as patients*. Bless you all - bigtime!

Patients were my main source of jokes. Most were truly appreciated, and I knew who would bring them in for me. Johnny Cleveland was a professional entertainer (read about him in *PATIENTS FROM HEAVEN - and Other Places!* Johnny did not come from the other place!). He *always* had a new, clean joke for me. So did Roly Lond. But I always braced myself when a chap gave a furtive grin, and said, "Now your nurse is out of the room, have you heard the one about...?" These days I hear few jokes, but a couple of good friends at our Norwich Full Gospel Businessmen's Fellowship, sometimes have me creased up. Thank you Bob Waters and Cliff Pain.

Proofreaders are invaluable. If readers could see the first draft of one of my books, they might be surprised to know that I actually passed English Language and English Literature at GCE Ordinary Level. But that was before the day of word processors and computers, where errors called *typos* creep in unnoticed. So I read the manuscript through several times myself. Then Wonder Woman, wife Wendy reads it, and turns in a whole crop of further mistakes, misprints, repetitions, examples of poor grammar and misspellings. Having checked the manuscripts at home, Barry Harvey takes over. Maestro of proofreaders, this man goes on to identify and list several pages of unnoticed and unwanted errors of grammar, spelling - and of pure fact. Also with this book, our hero suggested a change in the *structure* – which proved quite valuable. Thank you so much Barry; your meticulous scanning of my manuscripts is appreciated immensely. Linda Lyon and Tina Webber are not just good friends of ours – they are readers. I am indebted to each of them for reading through the manuscript of this book and giving me their honest opinion. It was so very helpful.

Derek Blois is an amazing man. He had a design studio in the town where I practised, but his influence went way beyond our community or county – or country. He was responsible for marketing *Spring Harvest*, a Christian convention hosting tens of thousands of, largely, young Christians. And so much more. Derek has designed the cover of each of my books, and has yet again surpassed my expectations. Thank you so much. In fact, Derek has become something of a celebrity artist in recent years, and deservedly so. His work can be viewed at the *PictureCraft Gallery & Exhibition Centre*, in Holt, Norfolk, and online at *www.picturecraftgallery.co.uk/derek-blois-bahons-aiea/*

My four daughters are a continual joy to me, and always have been. We love being together, and have innumerable treasured memories. They were as excited as I was when my first book was published some years ago, and continue to cheer me on as book number five hits the booksellers. Furthermore, they still laugh at my jokes. Sarah, Rachel, Naomi and Deborah - I love you so much, and you are in my thoughts every day. You are superstars - the best!

Wendy - Wonder Woman, as she is known to so many of our friends and acquaintances! I had been ditched in August 2001 and was alone again, wondering what sort of future lay before me. I enjoy female company and I enjoy restaurants, and back in early 2002, I was enjoying a lot of each.

One day I was in church and a lady went forward and spoke for a few minutes through the microphone on the platform. I had known her for eighteen years, perhaps, yet never really spoken to her. So that evening I did, telephoning to ask what she had said that morning, in more detail - and inviting her out for dinner. Our first date was 'OK', but nothing special. However, over the following months, I came to love that lady - and married her. Today, we feel we are a team like no other team. We host hundreds of people in our home, and travel widely to speak at all sorts of meetings in all sorts of places. I think she is amazing - so encouraging, inclusive, tolerant, hospitable, romantic... I can hardly believe how in love I am with my amazing wife. Thank you, Jesus, for bringing us together, and for all you are to us. And, of course, she proofreads my manuscripts and encourages enormously.

Although this is mainly a secular book, I want to acknowledge the God who changed my life back in 1965, filled me with his Spirit in 1967, and restored me as he forgave a major mess up in the early 1980s. Whilst only too aware of my own imperfections and inadequacies, I seek, by the grace of God, to put Jesus first in my life. We are told that if we give priority to seeking his kingdom, then everything else will fall into place (Matthew 6:33). I have found this to be true and will never cease to praise him.

Finally, there are you, my readers. Where would I be without you? Thank you for buying and reading this book, and presumably getting this far. So many of you are amazingly loyal, and I am grateful to those who write to me, email with kind words, and recommend my books to your friends. May God bless you richly indeed.

CURIOUS PEOPLE, HUMOROUS HAPPENINGS, CROWNS OF GLORY

A DENTIST'S STORY

by Barrie Lawrence
Published by Grosvenor House Publishing (2014)

After-dinner speaker Barrie Lawrence has been making people laugh - *really* laugh - for years. Now it's your turn to hear his unbelievably funny, sometimes poignant stories from dental school, surgery and life. How did a pet frog lead to a successful career of seven dental surgeries and a bookshop? And of course, he was a student during those years known as the 'Swinging Sixties!'

How can a filling take five hours to complete, and why did one of the lecturers at his dental school describe Barrie qualifying as 'like letting a monkey loose with a pistol'?

Read of some of those incidents and memories that have been making people smile for years when Barrie has been engaged in after-dinner speaking – or simply to the local Women's Institute. Do families of five really share just one toothbrush between them? Do that many dentures sail away down the toilet every winter? Have you ever come across people who share a set of false teeth between them?

But something happened while Barrie was training at the London Hospital – something that was even more important than training as a dentist!

You'll laugh, you'll cry, and most important of all, you will be inspired.

Available from www.amazon.co.uk *in the United Kingdom, and* www.amazon.com *in North America, and from all good bookshops*

* * *

"A refreshing delight. The author succeeds in maintaining interest by careful selection of anecdotes combined with a light-hearted tone and appropriate pace. I would recommend this book to anybody... looking for something uncomplicated and entertaining."

British Dental Journal, *Review by T. Doshi, December 2014*

"An entertaining and encouraging read." **Network Norwich.**

PATIENTS FROM HEAVEN
– and other places!

By Barrie Lawrence
Published by Grosvenor House (2015)

Baron Goldfinger seemed to have stepped straight off the James Bond movie set, Tad the Pole caused the nurses to swoon, while Misty, the flirtatious American lady, suddenly vanished – probably murdered, said the police. These and dozens of other colourful characters walk across the pages of *Patients From Heaven – and Other Places!* During nearly forty years of practice in dental surgery, a wealth of fascinating personalities passed through his surgery. Some were from heaven - and some were from other places! Laugh, smile, gasp, cry, and simply be inspired as you read through these engaging stories from real life.

Available from www.amazon.co.uk *(UK),* www.amazon.com *(North America) and all good bookshops.*

* * *

"Barrie introduces us to some of the most memorable people he met in this lovely and engaging memoir, the follow-up of his well-received *A Dentist's Story*. This is a lively read – he has a real way with a tale that keeps you turning the pages. Barrie is a practising Christian, but he doesn't hit you over the head with it; only mentioning it 'as and when' to put his story into context. An enjoyable – and rather uplifting – read."

Eastern Daily Press, *Review by Trevor Heaton, June 2015*

The style of writing reflects Barrie's skill as an engaging and very humorous after dinner speaker. He starts with those (patients) that became friends, or had something that endeared them to him and his staff; others made them laugh, or simply left them feeling better.

How does he depict patients from the *Other Place*? His belief as a born-again Christian, he says, changed everything including the way he sees other people. Courteously, he also sees this category of people with emotions, maybe struggling with relationships or finance. Chapters like "Blue Murder, a Pink Ear, Bubbles and a Bad Smell", "Nice and Nasty" and "The Gift of the Gab" have to be read.

Barrie balances his stories with patient's perceptions about him, with one patient calling him "a dangerous man".

His previous title *"A Dentist's Story"* concluded with an appendix of dental jokes and this time there is an appendix of anecdotes concerning encounters with members of the police force. Chapters including "The Man in Black", "Idiot!", "The Insurance Fraud?" and "A Carnivorous Villain" leave the reader entertained and bursting with laughter.

This book can easily be read and savoured like a meal with many courses over a period or devoured in one long sitting. Ideal as a holiday read and to pass on.

Network Norwich, Review by Kevin Gotts, August 2015

Patients from Heaven brilliantly explores Barrie Lawrence's plethora of patient experiences and stories in an equally hilarious and tasteful manner. Being a dental professional exposes us to a vast array of patients providing a wide range of wonderful and not so wonderful memories. Barrie takes us on a journey through all the memorable patients he has seen and all the lessons he has learned, whilst also respecting patient confidentiality (and brilliantly using fictional names and clever puns). *Patients from heaven* is a delightful read.

British Dental Journal, December 2015, Issue 11. Reviewed by K. Mahmood

THERE MUST BE MORE
TO LIFE THAN THIS!

How to know the God of the Bible in Everyday Life

by Barrie Lawrence

Published by New Wine Press (2012)

Barrie writes in his own distinctive style of incidents in his life that can only be described as amazing coincidences – or acts of God!

Barrie sent a paperback book to a patient, as he thought it would be helpful. The patient's wife took it from the postman, panicked, and called the emergency services to say a bomb had just been delivered. Why? A lady Barrie had known several years earlier, was woken up in the night to hear the Lord say to her, "Pray for Barrie Lawrence." Years later she was amazed to find out just why! And there was the time when a teapot prevented Barrie from really enjoying life as it was meant to be. How could that be? And then again there was the time when he and his wife were called to a school to heal a boy with a deformed arm – and the whole class were waiting to watch the miracle.

Not without humour, Barrie writes of the ways *he* has been challenged on various occasions in his life, of his successes and his failures. It's OK to laugh at him at times, because he does so himself, but you may also want to weep with him as he opens his heart about coping with difficulties and heartbreaks. Above all, it is an inspiring book that seeks to lift the reader onto a higher plane in life.

The first half of the book, part one, comprises fifteen short chapters of true stories from Barrie's own life, while part two has a clear message – it's happened to me and it can happen to you. In fact, part two is a reader-friendly guide to help anyone to come to know the God who we read about in the Bible.

If there are times when you think to yourself, "There must be more to life than this," then this book is a *must-read* for you!

Available from www.amazon.co.uk *and all good bookshops.*

A brilliant book by Barrie Lawrence. For anyone asking, '**Is there more to life than this?**' the author reveals a resounding 'Yes'. He shares his own journey of faith with refreshing candour – and then shows how the reader can experience Life with a capital L.

Michael Wiltshire, author and journalist, and a director of FGB, the world's largest fellowship for Christian businessmen.

Barrie Lawrence writes for Christians who compare their uneventful lives to all the excitement they read about in the Bible, and want to experience more of the latter. He shares some of his life story from nearly 50 years of being a Christian before pointing his readers to pointers for experiencing God for themselves. A sincere and candid little book.

Christianity Magazine, April 2013

Barrie has an infectious enthusiasm about the things of God and a burning desire to share them with others. The underlying theme is the breaking in of the supernatural to ordinary lives, and the importance of experiencing as well as believing.

Network Norwich, February 2013

THE CURIOUS CASE OF
THE CONSTIPATED CAT –

and Other True Stories of Answered Prayer

by Barrie Lawrence
Published by Grosvenor House (2016)

A terminally constipated pussy cat, two frozen shoulders, a man with a broken arm, a boy with a deformed arm, broken relationships, work overload, lost at night in a foreign city, irritable bowel, Crohn's Disease, financial challenges, wanting a husband, wanting a wife, not wanting divorce... All these needs were met after prayer. Coincidences? Psychosomatic? Don't be so silly. Come on - get real! Barrie and Wendy Lawrence, two very ordinary people, say, "If He can do it for us, then He can do it for you." Is anything too hard for the LORD? Get a realistic, meaningful relationship with the King of kings, and be amazed at what He can do in *your* life. This book is all about JESUS!

Available from www.amazon.co.uk *in the United Kingdom, and* www.amazon.com *in North America, and from all good bookshops*

* * *

"Feel your faith rise as you read these stories of answered prayer - faith to reach out to the God who can meet *your* need too."

Don Double, Evangelist and Founder, Good News Crusade.

"It's not the most conventional title for a Christian book. But then Barrie Lawrence is no average author. *The Curious Case of the Constipated Cat and Other True Stories of Answered Prayer* is the fourth book penned by Mr. Lawrence, a dentist, author and speaker. The book is different because not many 'religious books' are written in (his) style. Well, look at the title for a start! It is a collection of true stories of answered prayer, ranging from a cat being cured of constipation, and fog suddenly lifting so a flight could take off, to a troubled marriage being saved"

Eastern Daily Press *Review by Ian Clarke, 26ᵗʰ March 2016*

Good storytellers attract and engage their audiences quickly. Barrie, known for his straightforward, compelling and non-jargon style – refreshing for many Christians - has compiled interesting and often entertaining stories of a constipated cat, a boy with a deformed arm, an angel in Venice, a romance restored, an irritable bowel and many more relating to answered prayer. He playfully ends some accounts with a view that some people would consider the outcomes as "it's a coincidence, or maybe psychosomatic."

Enthusiasm underpins Barrie's approach to life. To find out more about the cat and as a helpful guide to answered prayer, do buy the book.

Network Norwich. *Review by Kevin Gotts*

I've just finished a great little book on prayer which I would heartily recommend. *The Curious Case of the Constipated Cat – and Other True Stories of Answered Prayer* was just the easy encouraging read I needed. In his light-hearted way, Barrie recounts various accounts of answered prayer before explaining our relationship with our Heavenly Father, and how we communicate with Him. Using the outline of the Lord's Prayer, Barrie highlights some basics about our relationship with our Heavenly Father and appropriate attitudes to develop an effective prayer life. Some great gems and interesting illustrations on how to approach some of the complexities of faith.

*Editorial in **Three-in-One** magazine of the Christian Dental Fellowship, by Victoria Rushton, President. Summer 2016*

Lightning Source UK Ltd.
Milton Keynes UK
UKOW04f1053310817
308315UK00001B/16/P